# Oh No, Not Another 'Growth' Opportunity!

## An Inspirational Cancer Journey With Humor, Heart, and Healing

Janet Jacobsen

Published by
Growth-Ink Publishing
4025 State Street, #9
Santa Barbara, CA 93110


Cover design by Janet Jacobsen

Cover graphics by Thomas Biesanz


Printed in the United States of America

ISBN NUMBER: 978-0-9799636-4-3

## WHAT PEOPLE ARE SAYING

The following are responses to the essays contained in this book, which were sent out as newsletters chronicling a 2 1/2 year cancer journey.

~~~~~~

"What a wonderful essay! So clear and deep, an inner ocean of knowing –beautiful!"  —Mary-Margaret Moore
Author of *I Come As A Brother (A Bartholomew book)*

"You are facing into this challenge with such audacity, courage, and humor. Your writing so eloquently of your experience is a tremendous gift. What a fabulous set of insights and learnings expressed in a right-now way."  —Kathlyn Hendricks, Co-Author of *Conscious Loving*

"I love and am deeply touched by your insights. The gifts that you're giving me are amazing. I have often wondered how people feel when they go through the 'cancer experience.' Now I know how a very aware person feels, and how they handle it."  —Pamala Oslie
Author of *Life Colors*

"I am delighted each time I read another one of your essays–so rich–so inspiring–so reminding!"  —Dale Figtree
Author of *Beyond Cancer Treatment*

"In my whole life I have never known anyone who so completely embraced cancer as a way to climb to such an incredible level of consciousness. I feel so touched and enlightened by the way you live your life, and inspire all of us to live too!"  —Kate Ludeman
Co-Author of *The Corporate Mystic*

"Beautiful words! I just wish the whole world could be reading these writings…they are so healing and speak to me on many levels."  —Diana Chapman, Advisor to Exceptional Leaders

"I loved this! I have uterine cancer too. I don't know what the future will be for me, but your words help me to look forward with hope and optimism!"  —Jackie McQueeney

"Beautiful…stunningly beautiful! Feeling a huge wave of gratitude for the journey you're on, and your choice to share it all with such transparency and heart."  —Corinna Bloom, Life Coach

"What an inspirational message. I enjoyed it and smiled often while reading it, and actually said 'wow' out loud twice."  —Walter Witkowski, Teacher

"You write so beautifully. Each essay captivates me with its rawness, honesty, insight and inspiration. I gain so much from each one of them and apply it to my own journey with cancer." —Martha McVay

"It is such a gift to share this journey with you, but more than that, to see the transformative opportunities that you experience and share as a result of the diagnosis." —Barbara Monett, Psychotherapist

"As always, I love the insightfulness and consciousness you bring to your journey and then share with others." —Melanie Brown
Conscious Cancer Coach

"Your writing is so crystal clear. Thank you for enlightening me on so many subjects, written in such an eloquently deep, yet humorous pen." —David Biesanz, Teacher

"I love your writing! This is really rich stuff." —PatriciaSelbert
Author of *The House of Six Doors*

"I can't begin to express how moving and inspirational your essays have been. Your voice is beautiful and clear, and I find myself crying, and at the same time feeling joyful when I read your amazing essence expression. Thank you for the awakening that your writing is inspiring in me." —Dru Zuretti

"Your writing is so beautiful, so powerful, so astonishing, so helpful, so inspiring, so moving, so adorable, so resonant! Thank you, thank you!" —Christopher Pilafian , Choreographer

"I receive healing from you each time I read what you have to say." —Grace Caitlyn, Life Coach

"I enjoy every one of your essays and I'm thoroughly inspired by your messages. You're a remarkable person, with depth and pluck – a fabulously clever writer." —J'Nelle Holland

"Somehow, miraculously through this emotional roller coaster you've been on, you are able to share yourself on such an incredibly deep level." —Amanda Mardon

"I love reading amazing stories of people who overcome health challenges, like cancer, with positive energy! Your positive energy and thoughts continue to be an inspiration." —Carol Sauceda

# TABLE OF CONTENTS

# ACKNOWLEDGEMENTS

I am grateful for my husband, Tom Biesanz, whose depth of spirit and lightness of soul have blessed my life with such joy. It is a great pleasure to spend each day with you, laughing, learning, and growing together. Thank you for being my spiritual partner and playmate in this life. It just keeps getting better and better.

I appreciate the many family and friends who love, support, and encourage me to be my authentic self and express that in writing. A true friend is someone who knows everything about you and loves you anyway. Thank you for loving and welcoming my warts and all self.

I deeply value the many people who have been following my journey through my newsletters. It is such an honor that you are allowing me to share with you all that I'm learning along the way. Thank you!

*This book is dedicated to all of us who are experiencing growth opportunities in our lives. May we learn and grow with ease and flow, and find our place in a state of grace.*

# INTRODUCTION:
# LEMONS INTO LEMONADE

By the time I turned 60 I had gotten to a place in my life where I was the happiest I'd ever been. I was with my long-awaited soul mate and we were enjoying a deep, rich, fun relationship of ten years. I had wonderful friends, ate healthy food, processed my emotions, and connected with my spirit on a regular basis. I'd conquered my life-long issues of low self-esteem and fear of intimacy and was finally living a life filled with joy and love. I felt at peace with myself. I thought I was home free. That's why I was shocked when I was diagnosed with uterine cancer! What the…?!

As someone on a personal growth path, I believe that life is all about learning and growing and evolving our souls. After I recovered from the shock of the diagnosis, I could appreciate that this cancer growth was a growth opportunity and I was determined to get the most growth I could from it! It was also an opportunity to share with others a treasure trove of learning I'd gathered along the way that could be helpful with any kind of life challenge.

I'd always wanted to do inspirational writing and often told myself that someday I would write. Cancer kicked my 'someday' into 'write now!' I started writing essays chronicling my journey and e-mailing them out in a newsletter. I was thrilled that people told me they were inspired and learning from my journey. I was finally fulfilling my dream of being of service to others with my writing.

I felt that this was the missing piece. I had been doing the same work as an artist and craftsperson for 25 years and felt stagnant and bored with it. Now I was doing the inspirational writing that my soul longed to do. Once again,

I thought I was home free…and once again, cancer came a calling! A year after my hysterectomy to remove the cancer, a year in which I was eating raw food, drinking wheat grass juice, confronting my fears, fulfilling my life purpose, and learning to value each moment, a tumor the size of a lemon had grown in my pelvic area! "Oh no! Not another 'growth' opportunity!"

Life had given me a lemon—a really sour, potentially lethal lemon! My oncologist recommended chemo and radiation treatment, and even with that grueling regimen, he gave me low odds of survival. Yikes! Why was this happening?! I was facing death, a painful death at that, and I was stunned.

After I recovered from this new shock, I plunged even deeper into this 'growth' opportunity, determined to turn this sour lemon into sweet lemonade. If my time was short, I wanted to get as much juice as I could out of it—to live, learn, grow, and share fully.

This book contains the inspirational essays I wrote on my journey, presented in the sequence they were written. With humor, heart, and raw honesty, it reveals the gold I've mined along the way, as well as the emotional and spiritual practices, and the diet, supplements, and alternative treatments I'm doing that I believe have extended my life, and maybe even cured my cancer. It is a journey of healing on many levels.

This has been, and continues to be, a soul-stirring, heart-opening, mind-blowing growth experience! Thank you for coming along with me on this adventure! As you read my story, may you be inspired, touched, informed, and, at times, even amused! Yes, it's true…we can find humor in ANYTHING!

# 1

## WHAT WANTS TO BE BORN?
(February 25, 2009)

I've been thinking about birth lately. My 60th birthday is about a week away and I'm choosing to see it as a time of rebirth. I've been wondering, what wants to be born into my next decade on planet earth?

When I turned 50 I began a new life with Tom, my life partner. I had been single most of my life so it was a major shift for me. I deeply desired it and that is the beginning of any birth process. First there was *desire*, then being able to *conceive* that it was possible, then *labor* (taking action), and finally the Universe *delivered* to me a beautiful, bouncing babe of a man named Tom and a healthy, happy, thriving relationship that is now ten years old! As the big 6-0 approaches, I'm wondering, what wants to be born next?

Another reason I've been thinking about birth is because something has been growing in my uterus. Ultrasounds have shown that it has doubled in size in this past year filling the uterine cavity. I appreciated the symbolism of something growing in my uterus and something new wanting to be born into my life. I was hoping it was just a benign polyp, as it appeared to be when I had it checked out a year ago.

On Friday my doctor did a procedure called a hysteroscopy where he went into my uterus with a tiny camera to determine what was growing. He took out a piece to biopsy. He said it appeared fluffy, like a cotton ball, and was 99% certain that it was cancerous. I was stunned! Yesterday he confirmed that it is cancer. That was not what

I wanted to hear. This seemed like something to be borne, instead of a new life being born.

When I was first told that I should have this hysteroscopic procedure, I wanted to put it off because it was expensive and invasive. I wanted to try alternative methods instead. But persistent thoughts about my mother (who is deceased) kept hovering in my mind, nudging me to take medical action. That's something I know she would want me to do. I finally decided to make an appointment with the doctor and the date for the consult just happened to land on my mother's birthday!

Since hearing that it was cancer I've been feeling contractions of fear, and urges to curl up into the fetal position. Yet awareness tells me that contractions precede birth—contractions lead to expansions. I know from experience that any feeling that is fully felt and experienced always leads to expansion. So, just like in childbirth, I've been breathing into these fear contractions, feeling them fully, allowing them to be here. Eventually that has brought me to a more expanded place.

In that expanded place a strong awareness and desire came to me—I know what wants to be born into my life—I want to write! I want to be of service by sharing my living, loving, laughing, and learning about life's luminous (and sometimes lousy) lessons. I want to put my writing into a form and send it out into the world. That's the reason for this birth announcement; I have birthed my first newsletter and am sending it out into the world!

I didn't think I'd ever get cancer. I have always been terrified of the thought of cancer. I still can't quite believe it. I didn't think I'd be giving birth to my entire uterus (via hysterectomy)! Some babies **really** suck, and this is one big, sucky turn of events. But even though I am sometimes a big baby full of fears and tears, I also have a big brave, nurturing soul that embraces all that shows up. I know that whatever happens in my life is ALL about my soul growth. I intend to cultivate the most growth I can from this experience, and all the other life lessons that come my way.

I'd like to leave you with this question: What contractions are you feeling in your life? What gestating dream of yours is ready to be born? I'm wishing you a joyful "birth" and that your contractions shift easefully into expansion!

**2**

# WAKING UP WITH FEAR
(March 5, 2009)

Today is my 60<sup>th</sup> birthday! It's more like my *re*birth day. My recent diagnosis of uterine cancer has grabbed me by the ankles, turned me upside down, and spanked me vividly alive! The familiar day-to-day sameness that lulled me to sleep is upended as life sings me awake with a rousing lull-*goodbye* song. I open my birthday Present, fully here and now, brand spanking new…and scared.

I have been waking up with fear. There's a lot of that going around right now. The country has been turned upside down, swatted on its bottom, and startled awake as the economy quakes on shaky ground. Maybe some of you are feeling fear right now in your lives about an illness, or the loss of a relationship, loved one, job, or home?

I'm experiencing that fear has a life of its own. It is primal, survival-oriented and hardwired. It will not release its grip easily. Like a tightly wound rosebud that cannot be forced open, it must be allowed to gently unfold. Fear is a compelling force we can use to help us unfold fully into this Present Moment and transform scared energy into sacred energy. I'd like to share with you this process of 'face, embrace, and replace' that is helping me use fear to Wake Up and smell the roses.

AWARENESS
I awake in the grip of fear and say, "I feel scared."

Acknowledging and naming the feeling is the first step. I generate curiosity about the fear. Where do I feel it? It is a clenching tension that feels like a boa constrictor wrapped around my entire body, squeezing most tightly around my throat, chest, solar plexus, and stomach. I notice my breathing is barely there. This act of witnessing has invited in another level of consciousness. Now there is fear and there is awareness. I spontaneously begin to breathe more fully.

## SELF-COMPASSION

I notice that this fear is like a child who is suffering. I cradle the fear. I place my hands on my throat and my heart, and comfort the fear. "Hello fear. You are welcome here. It's okay to feel scared. I'm sorry you are suffering. I know this is difficult. I understand." I place my hands over my uterus. "I love you. I'm sorry you are sick. I am so sorry to be losing you." I cry. It is a *good cry, good grief,* releasing stress; the tears carry out the stress hormone cortisol. Now there is sadness, fear, awareness, compassion and slow gentle breaths.

## COMPASSION FOR OTHERS

Tonglen is a Buddhist meditation practice in which I breathe in my fear and sadness and feel it fully and I breathe out sending love and compassion to everyone who is feeling that same pain. Breathing in, I feel sad and scared—breathing out, I send love to others who are feeling sad and scared.

I repeat this for several minutes. This creates a feeling of love and connection to others. It's also a comfort to know that I'm not alone in this fear, others are feeling it too. Now, in this expanding field, there is sadness, fear, awareness, and compassion for myself and for others. My painful feelings are subsiding. I still feel them, but I am feeling serenity as well. I rest in a nurturing loving energy that embraces it all.

TRUST, ACCEPTANCE, GRATITUDE—(TAG).
My feelings have calmed enough that I am now open to a higher awareness. I generate the energy of trust, acceptance and gratitude by affirming:

I **Trust** that I am loved, guided and watched over. I trust that things happen for a reason. I trust that my life is purposeful. I trust that everything will work out.

I **Accept** that this is what's happening. It is what is. I breathe and allow it to be. This moment is perfect just as it is. I surrender to it. I become one with it.

I feel **Gratitude** for the many blessings in my life: my loving friends and family, my fellow journeyers and learning buddies, my wonderful husband Tom. I am grateful for this opportunity to cultivate more awareness, love, trust, and acceptance in my life. I am grateful that I remember that this is what is most important to me. I am grateful that I am awake. I am grateful to fear for waking me up.

What challenges are waking you up? What feelings of yours want to be faced, embraced, and replaced? Taking time to stop and smell the roses and feel the feelings allows them to unfold into the full bloom of Present Moment consciousness; makes sweet sense to me. I love getting roses on my birthday!

# 3

# BRIGHT LIGHT, DARK SHADOWS
(March 11, 2009)

Seven months ago my appendix burst and was removed. Now my cancerous uterus is about to be removed. What's up down there? My internal organs are jumping ship! I can't help but wonder, have I done something wrong? I'd always thought that this couldn't happen to me. I take good care of myself, I eat healthy, don't drink alcohol or smoke, I exercise, ingest a fistful of vitamins every day, express my thoughts and feelings, connect with my spirit, and have loving relationships. I thought I was safe. Now a part of me feels like I have failed in some way.

Cancer is such a violent thing to have inside me. It is something shadowy, dark and dangerous that will kill me unless I kill it first. This has stirred up my painful old core belief which says, "I didn't just do something wrong, I *am* something wrong; I am fundamentally damaged; and bad things happen to me because I'm bad." The pain of that core belief has set me on a spiritual path for the last 40 years. I have read a great multitude of spiritual and personal growth books and attended more workshops that you can shake a talking stick at. I have grown and healed tremendously. Yet still…cancer.

Feeling sad and disappointed, I lay in my husband Tom's arms, crying, "I am flawed. After all these years and all the work I've done on myself, I am still deeply flawed." Tom smiled and said, "Me too." We both laugh. I have done something right to have this blessing of a man in my life! He has helped me put the *fun* into *fun*damentally flawed. Just looking at him reminds me that there is much light in my life now. And, there are still shadows. Tom says, "The brighter the light is the more clearly defined the shadows are." Yes. The light is shining brightly in my life and I'm seeing my shadows very clearly. That is a good thing.

One way the Universe very clearly reveals my shadows to me is through the people in my life. They are wonderful mirrors—I can clearly see in *them* how they are defensive, judgmental, victimy, and oblivious to it (as much as I try to point it out to them!) These people can be irritating to be around. When I try to remove them from my life, they just keep showing up in different bodies with new names!

My shadows are clearly defined and they are clearly following me! Wherever I go, there I am. I'm learning that if it's in my life, it's in me. More importantly, I'm seeing that it's all about Love. These shadows keep showing up to be faced, accepted and loved in me, and in those who are mirroring me.

I am facing and accepting that I will never be perfect. I lose my temper, I stress out, and I like to indulge in a fine whine now and then. I'm learning to shine the light on all that I am, to love myself As Is, warts and all...and now, cancer and all.

Life is not about being perfect—it's about being whole. As Carl Jung said, "I'd rather be whole than good." Loving ALL of me is loving myself whole (minus a few body parts). I feel compassion for that part of us that gets lost in the shadows. I feel such love and appreciation for how we keep striving for the light, sometimes floundering towards the light. How brave we all are to be here on this journey on planet earth, fallible, flawed and perfectly imperfect.

We are right where we need to be. This moment is perfect just as it is. This cancer is perfect just as it is. Healing and learning are happening. My dearly departing body parts are leaving me with this wonderful parting gift—the reminder to welcome every part and parcel of me to the party. I welcome cancer as my teacher.

Are there people and circumstances that keep showing up in your life, shadowing you? You haven't done anything wrong. Life is simply reflecting back to you what wants to be faced and embraced.

**4**

# THE WONDERFUL WISDOM OF 'IS'
(March 18, 2009)

The mind is like a crazed acrobat, tumbling from thought to thought, leaping to conclusions. I've been witnessing my mind tumbling about trying to figure things out and find answers. It wants to know, how did I end up with uterine cancer? Could it be the occasional sugar? The dairy? The aspartame? Or is it because I'm uptight; or more accurately, *down*tight? (as in anal retentive.) Did I block the flow of chi down there? Or could it be that my laptop sitting on my lap is frying my innards, doing the lap dance of death!?

Who knows why things happen. The only thing I can know for certain is this…it happened. It is what it is. I am open to learning and seeing my part in things, but I am becoming more interested right now in learning the fine art of acceptance. Now is all there is, and this is what's Now. There is no right or wrong—just Isness. Buddha called this state Tatata. I want to live in this state. I am packing up my baggage and moving to Tatata, the golden state of harmony with what IS.

I'm leaving behind self-blame, trying to figure things out, and regret. They are not useful. Much suffering is caused by resisting what is happening. It's like trying to resist a tornado—it's only going to mess you up! When I accept what is happening and say, "Oh, this is interesting. I wonder what I can learn from it?" I come into harmony with it and it delivers me to the wonderful land of IS. When I'm focused on learning and growing, then every experience is perfect.

This morning I had my long-awaited appointment with the oncologist to consult and set the date for my hysterectomy. When I got there they told me that they didn't have my name down! At first I cried; it felt good to release the tension. Then, I could feel the downward vortex, the circling the drain energy, wanting to *poor me* down the drain, wanting to blame and complain. Noticing this, I took a breath and said to myself, "It's okay to feel scared and angry. Let yourself feel it." I began to breathe more easily. Allowing these feelings to be present helped return me to the state of IS. It is what it IS. Breathe. Accept. This moment is perfect just as it is. (Fortunately, they rescheduled me for later in the day.)

The mind always wants to know, "Is this a good thing? Is this a bad thing?" Byron Katie has written that when people used to say "Namaste" to her, she delightedly thought they were saying "No mistake". My appendix burst seven months ago. That could have killed me...or it could have saved my life. The CT scan they did for my appendix showed that my uterus was abnormal. That led to the discovery of the uterine cancer.

My brother found out he had an inoperable brain aneurysm. He thought his life was over. It had just begun! He quit his job, bought a sailboat and now, 8 years later, is enjoying life on his boat sailing the Caribbean Islands, thriving and living his dream. "Just when the caterpillar thought its life was over, it became a butterfly."

My husband Tom is cultivating rich soil in his garden plot. It contains compost from rotted produce and horse manure. He treats these ingredients like precious gold. He knows they will help his garden grow the most nutritious, delicious food. Cancer has composted a rich and fertile soil for me, from which is sprouting creativity, inspiration, and learning. (It's a fertile time or it's a shitty time; same substance, different attitude).

The best part about being in harmony with what is, it hooks me up with the Universal flow. Once I am in the energy of acceptance, I am in a state of grace where things I need flow to me easily, and everything works out better than I could imagine. Rich gifts are coming my way: the love of family and friends, the best doctors and nurses, financial assistance, and powerful learning and healing on a deep level. Open is open—when I let go of resistance and open to what is, I am open to receive love, guidance and miracles.

Brick by golden brick I am building my home base in Tatata. I sometimes take little side trips to Self-Pity City (my old home town), and occasionally I am swept up in little cyclones of anger, sadness and fear. Accepting what is happening includes accepting all the feelings that come up about it. These feelings are like bulls in a pen, snorting and pawing the ground; when they are accepted as part of what Is and allowed to be, then the gate opens, freeing them to enter the big spacious field of awareness, where eventually they calm down and become One with the field. "Out beyond rightdoing and wrongdoing, there is a field; I'll meet you there." -(Rumi)  Right Here and Now there is a field of awareness where everything is welcome; there's plenty of room for ALL that shows up.

Are you living in the golden state of Tatata? It is a beautiful, spacious place to live. (And it's so much fun saying Tatata!)  To get there, just click your heels together, take deep, slow breaths of acceptance and say, "There's no place like Here. There's no place like Now." That will always bring you back Home again.

# 5

# MR. TOAD'S WILD ELEVATOR RIDE
(March 25, 2009)

A friend said to me recently, "You are on Mr. Toad's wild ride, and you're managing to enjoy the scenery." That made me smile. It *has* been a wild ride, but I'm experiencing it more like a wild elevator ride that goes up and down, and every floor has a different view. The first floor is a limited ego's eye view; the top floor is an expansive eagle's eye view.

Sometimes my elevator doesn't go all the way to the top; but when it does I can see the big picture. I can see how everything fits together perfectly. I can see how I am connected to it all.

When my buttons are pushed I often descend to the lower floors. Going down...THUMP! On the bottom floor there is worry, 'what ifs', 'whys', regrets, blame, danger, drama, duality, me versus them. On the bottom floor I am in the thick of it all.

Yesterday my elevator plummeted to the bottom floor. My sister told me that she was examined by her gynecologist this week, who was concerned about some unusual bleeding. The doctor right then and there in the office took a sample from her uterus to biopsy, just like that! Her doctor said under her breath that that is what my doctor should have done over a year ago when the abnormalities first came to his attention.

When I hear this I am stunned! My elevator crashes to the bottom floor! 'Whys' and 'what ifs' rush in. Why didn't they biopsy mine a year ago? (They did ultrasounds instead, which showed an apparently benign polyp, so nothing else was done.) What if it has spread? What if I have to suffer through chemo and radiation? What if I die because they didn't do the biopsy right away?

A flood of tears and fears and old pain bodies enter the scene saying, "The world is unsafe, people can't be trusted, I am in danger!" Anger rages on board. "They should've done it differently!" A girl named Sue stomps in, pumping her fist, chanting, "Sue, sue, sue the incompetents!" The elevator is getting very crowded!

Fortunately there is room for one more…my Compassionate Witness. She holds the space for everyone who shows up. She encourages good ventilation by saying, "It's ok to feel angry, sad and scared. Let yourself feel it. Feel it deeply. I will hold you." She does not try to tell me, "This moment is perfect just as it is." This is not a time or place for that. This is a time to BE where I'm at, in the thick of it, feeling it fully, shining the light of awareness on it.

I know from experience that if I try to rise above my feelings, that just positions me better for them to bite me in the butt! These feelings deserve to be heard and honored. If they are not, then they take up permanent residence on the bottom floor, spinning round and round in 'ain't it awful' stories, like a dog chasing its tale of woe. My elevator was stuck on the bottom floor for many years, until my Compassionate Witness came to live with me.

When I rest and release in this spacious loving awareness, I am naturally elevated to a higher perspective. Going up…I begin to get glimpses of how I collaborated with how it was done and the decisions that were made; I had been happy to minimize the abnormality and make it all go away. I can also see my doctor more clearly as someone who was caring and concerned, not a bad person out to hurt me.

My elevator ascends higher and I can see how on the

lower floors my mind's tendency is to seize on the 'what should've been's' of past and 'what ifs' of the future. From this elevated vantage point I am aware that there is only NOW. Right now is all there is and right now I am fine. I am more than fine. I am experiencing a treasure of learning and inspiration, as well as the great joy of writing and sharing my experience. If this had been nipped in the bud a year ago, would I be having such a rich, full-bloomed experience now?

I am seeing how it is perfect that this is bringing up my pain bodies; on the lower floors they are a torment, but elevated in awareness they become pain buddies, here to help me heal deeply imprinted fear and trust issues. I can see this is the healing that is most important; healing the belief that the world is unfriendly and I am its victim; loosening my ego's tenacious grip on feeling wronged; learning to forgive and let it go. It has been said that the highest form of forgiveness is being able to say, "Thank you *for giving* me this experience."

Right now, as I am peacefully perched on the top floor, I can see how it all fits together. Now I can hear and let in these words, "This moment is perfect just as it is." From this higher view I see and know that I am One with it all.

I also know that I will continue to ride the elevator up and down, but with my Compassionate Witness along, I am enjoying the scenery. There is no good or bad, right or wrong experience. There is just being with it with curiosity, compassion and a willingness to learn from it all. That always elevates me to the top floor.

*"Just go into the room and put one chair in the center.*
*Take the seat in the center of the room, open the door*
*and windows, and see who comes to visit.*
*You will witness all kinds of scenes and actors,*
*all kinds of temptations and stories, everything imaginable.*

*Your only job is to stay in your seat.*
*You will see it all arise and pass, and out of this—*
*wisdom and understanding will come."* -Achaan Chan

What is the view from your elevator right now? I hope that your Compassionate Witness is by your side helping you enjoy the scenery on your wild, wonderful, wisdom-gathering ride!

# 6

## STEP BY STEP, COURAGE
(April 1, 2009)

I walked into the hospital on Monday morning for my surgery, trembling like a dog walking into the vets. I put one foot in front of the other, and one step at a time, one breath at a time, I got through it!

I've always been afraid of hospitals and the idea of surgery. In the past I thought if I had to choose between hospitalization and death, I would choose death. I didn't think I had it in me to be able to handle it. But I am handling it. I am braver than I thought!

Cancer has been one of my worst fears. Over the years I've taken all kinds of anti-cancer measures (taking vitamin D, wearing sunscreen, eating broccoli, etc.), trying to keep it at bay. It's like I've been tiptoeing around a sleeping beast, trying not to wake it. Yet despite my best efforts, the beast has awakened!

A friend told me about someone she knew who had taken great care of his body, mind, and spirit; yet still he had a heart attack. He was sure it was a mistake and said, "Somewhere, there's a guy sitting in front of a TV watching wrestling, clutching a beer, with Cheetos dust floating down onto his big belly....and I HAD HIS HEART ATTACK!" We humans are so funny! We actually think we can control these things!

In early childhood I had a recurring dream in which I was walking into a field with other kids and they wanted to walk into the woods at the edge of the field. I was afraid of the big bad wolf in the woods, so I didn't go with them. I lay down on a picnic table in the open field by myself and thought I was safe; but when I opened my eyes, the wolf was there, right next to me, staring at me with sparkling flinty eyes! Even as a young child I was struck by the irony of it.

One way I've tried to keep the wolf from my door is by very carefully avoiding x-rays, not even wanting digital dental x-rays. When I had appendicitis a few months ago I was given a CT scan, which has 500 times more radiation than a normal x-ray! That wolf has a way of finding me no matter what I do! I've finally come to a place where I give up; I surrender; I throw up my hands; I let go of trying to control everything; I stop running.

I lie on my hospital bed pre-op, and in a field of awareness I take slow deep breaths and face the wolf. I get up close and curious about it's sharp teeth and claws. I look into its flinty eyes…and I discover…it is Fear in wolf's clothing! What I've feared is the biting discomfort of my throat-clutching, heart-pounding, gut-wrenching fear. FDR was right, "We have nothing to fear but fear itself." The *fear* of the cancer and the operation feels so much worse than the cancer itself.

I am now facing my fear, sitting with it, keeping it company, holding its hand, feeling compassion, allowing it to be here. I've heard two acronyms for FEAR: one is *Feel Everything And Recover*. The other is *F…k Everything And Run!* These are the different agendas of our ego and our spirit. Ego wants to run for the hills and be safe. Spirit wants to fly like an eagle as high as it can go, fully experiencing life, including fear.

When challenges befall me, my ego wails in a Mr. Bill whine, "Oh Noooooo. Not another learning opportunity!" My spirit says, "Oh Yeah! Another opportunity to grow! Bring it on!" My ego moans, "We are in deep doodoo!" My spirit exalts, "Rich soil, yay!" Ego scolds, "Now we've gone and done it...our fear has drawn the cancer to us!" Spirit exclaims, "Cool, cancer! It will help us come face to face with fear, feel it fully, and make friends with it!"

Who knows what our souls are up to—there's so much more going on than meets the eye—*WE* are so much more. When faced with the thing I most feared, I'm finding that I have more courage than I ever dreamed possible. My mind has been telling me that I'm "the biggest scaredy cat in the world." What I'm actually discovering is that I am someone who has the courage to be present with my worst fears, one breath at a time, one trembling foot in front of the other. Hand in hand with my Compassionate Witness, I am doing this! And if I can do this, anyone can!

We have more courage and spirit than we know. When we are tested, we somehow find the strength to soar with the eagles; no longer circling the drain, we are circling the sky!

# 7

# WAKE UP, YOU'RE ALIVE!
(April 8, 2009)

Tom's daughter Oakley came for a visit last week with her husband Len and their year-and-a-half-old son Arthur. Arthur was such a joy to observe; he sees life anew, with fresh eyes. As a train went by behind our house, he watched with wide-eyed wonder and exclaimed, "More choochoo!"

I am in pain from my hysterectomy. I wince as Tom helps me out of bed. Then I look at Tom and smile, grateful that he is in my life, helping me out of bed. I look at him the way Arthur looked at the train. My wide-open baby eyes drink him in. "More Tom!"

I lived alone for most of my life until I was 50 and met Tom. Ten years later he is still a surprise to me and I see him with fresh, grateful eyes…most of the time. Sometimes he and I will be busily buzzing through our day, and one of us will notice that and tap the other on the shoulder, look into their eyes and say, "Hello." Stopping in the middle of our busyness we become aware, "Oh, *you're* here." And then, "Oh, *I'm* here."

Since my diagnosis of uterine cancer and subsequent surgery, I have been experiencing life through baby eyes. It's much like lucid dreaming when you wake up *within* your dream and know that you're dreaming. This is lucid living; waking up in your life knowing that you're alive.

People who have had near-death experiences report that upon return to consciousness they see their life in vivid technicolor and have a renewed zest for life. Any life calamity can do the same. It rocks our world and we are jolted awake. "Wake up, you're alive!" In that way, our life calamities can be a great gift.

Brian Andreas, the creator of Story People, created a Story People drawing with the caption: "Most people don't know there are angels whose only job is to make sure you don't get too comfortable and fall asleep and miss your life." These wake-up angels are among us, cleverly disguised as calamities (and babies)! The brain is designed to categorize, habitualize, and go on automatic pilot. That's why it takes something new and out of the ordinary to wake us up to the Present Moment: something like a baby, a long-awaited love, or a calamity.

As the Titanic was sinking, the band was playing "Nearer My God to Thee", and the people on board were singing along. No doubt they were feeling vibrantly alive. I imagine the people in the lifeboats were feeling that same vivid aliveness. Voltaire said, "Life is a shipwreck, but we must not forget to sing in the lifeboats." We must not forget to sing and dance and be fully awake and alive in our life.

But not to worry…if we do forget, life will obligingly send us one of those angels to wake us up so that we don't miss our lives!

# 8

## REFRAMING AND RENAMING
(April 15, 2009)

My pathology report came back and showed that my nodes were clear. However, the cancer was more aggressive than they first thought and it had penetrated into two thirds of the uterine wall (making it Stage 1C, Grade 3). The doctor said there is a 25% risk of recurrence. I asked him, "Since I don't have a uterus anymore, where would the cancer go?" He said, "Anywhere."

That scared me—an image came to mind of marauding terrorist cells that had eluded the doctor's scalpel and were cunningly roaming my body, looking for a place to set up camp and wreak more havoc. Then I quickly reframed that. For one thing, I have a 75% chance that it **won't** recur. For another, I can see how the increased risk is perfect because it keeps me awake, on my toes, bright-eyed, bushy-tailed, and motivated to continue with the healing life changes I've made, like the vibrant diet, daily meditation, deep breathing, and enjoying my moment-to-moment game of TAG...continually coming back to Trust, Acceptance, and Gratitude. (TAG, I'm it. I choose what I want to focus on and generate.)

I am aware that words and images shape and color our world, they mold it like play doh. "Words cast spells, that's why they call it spelling." How we think of things and picture them creates a cellular response in our bodies. It is self-hypnosis. When hypnotized, our body can raise a blister if we're touched with an ice cube and told that it's a blazing hot coal.

Our thoughts can create heaven or hell, depending on where we're choosing to dwell. Thoughts create feelings of wellbeing, or of being stuck *in* a well. They also create chemicals in our body, such as feel-good endorphins, or the stress hormone cortisol. We literally are walking laboratories, and our thoughts are the chemists.

Words and images impact our immune system and ability to heal. A friend of Tom's told him that she had cancer a few years ago and was in two cancer support groups. There were people in the groups who had an attitude of being at war and battling their cancer. Other people had an attitude of wanting to learn and grow and explore what their cancer brought up for them. In her experience, those were the people who tended to survive, while the ones who were at war did not.

A friend told me that she doesn't use the word cancer, instead she calls it 'aberrant cells'. I've been playing with other names like waker-uppers, 'I' openers, shadows, fungi (some people believe that cancer is a fungus)…how about 'fun guy'? There's a woman who calls hers crazy, sexy cancer (and wrote a book with that title).

My cancer experience has opened my eyes big time in so many ways; therefore, I have decided to call it The Big See! I See the world with new eyes, big bright baby eyes. I See that I have more courage than I thought. I See the love of friends and family. I See that my life is purposeful and things happen for a reason. I See that our earth life is finite and our spirit is infinite. I See that it's all about love.

I invite all of you as you go through your day today to eavesdrop on yourselves. What thoughts are you dwelling on? What chemicals are you cooking up in your body lab? What is ready to be reframed and renamed in your life?

# 9

# OWNING YOUR MAGNIFICENCE
### (April 21, 2009)

A frumpy, middle-aged woman with bushy caterpillar eyebrows walked in nervous determination onto the stage. In front of millions of viewers of the TV show, Britain's Got Talent, she declared that her dream is to be a professional singer. People snickered and rolled their eyes. Then she began to sing in a beautiful, clear voice. People's jaws dropped, and a spontaneous standing ovation with thunderous applause erupted. Now over 100 million people have been moved, amazed, and inspired by Susan Boyle on Youtube.

I believe that one of the reasons this has touched so many people so profoundly is because deep down inside we know that we have within us our own version of jaw-dropping magnificence. Just like the Ugly Duckling, our beautiful swan essence exists, waiting to be owned and revealed.

Gay Hendricks says, "We are so busy trying to prove we're okay, we forget that we're magnificent." I believe that, like the Ugly Duckling, we are all on a hero's journey to discover our inherent magnificence. One of the challenges on our journey is that we misidentify ourselves as the Ugly Duckling and get lost in that image and stuck in that story. When we try to break free and be more than that, a critical inner voice berates us, saying, "Who do you think you are?" Yet there is a higher voice within urging us to remember, "Who do you KNOW you are?"

Sometimes a life challenge, such as a divorce, an illness, or a great loss, comes along to wake us up and help us remember who we really are. When first confronted with adversity, it can seem that life has turned on us; but we eventually find instead that it has turned us ON! It has turned on the big, bright, luminous light of our soul, igniting our courage, strength, and special abilities, reminding us that, like Susan Boyle, there is so much more to us than meets the eye.

I had planted a thought seed years ago that in my 60's I would be optimally healthy. I would be slender. I would be writing. I would be deeply connected with my spirit. Yet as the big 6-0 was just months away I found myself thirty pounds overweight and cozily nestled into the comfort of the familiar. I needed something to jolt me into a strong resolve for this life transformation, and I got it! (Life is so accommodating!)

As a result of my appendicitis and uterine cancer, something remarkable has happened…I saw something today that I haven't seen in years…my jaw line! When my appendicitis struck 9 months ago I completely lost my appetite! I ate very lightly for three months and lost 23 pounds! When the possibility of uterine cancer entered the scene a few months ago, I changed my diet even more, eating mostly raw foods, drinking wheat grass juice everyday, and cutting out all dairy and sugar. I lost seven more pounds.

The seed I had planted prior to turning 60 is now in full bloom. I feel more vibrantly healthy and alive than I have ever felt. I am loving my body (including my new scars, which I see as badges of courage). I am deeply connected with my spirit. And I am writing and sharing about it all with others!

My jaw drops as I see that this frumpy, complacent, middle-aged woman that I was just nine months ago has transformed into my Magnificent Kick-Ass Big Soul Self, doing the soul work that I came here to do!

Who do you KNOW you are? Have you owned and revealed your jaw-dropping magnificence?

## 10

## SWEET SOUL WHISPERS
(April 29, 2009)

I'm lying on my back and my cat Zeena is circling me; she wants to lay on my soft warm belly, as she usually does. "No," I say. I am guarding my belly; it is still sore from the hysterectomy, and vulnerable. I protect it like a mama bear protecting her cub from a mountain lion.

This girding of my belly is a familiar thing. I am often aware of a clenching tension in my belly. It makes sense to me that this stress would block the flow of energy, oxygen, life force, and chi, leaving me susceptible to health problems in that area.

I tell this to Tom and he says, "You use the word stress a lot. What do you mean by it?" "Hmm, good question." I tune into the feeling of stress. "It is really fear." "What do you mean by fear?" he asked. I close my eyes and feel into it more deeply. What I experience is that I am breathing shallowly and my belly is tight, contracted, armored, as if resisting. I see that it's all about protection. It is the opposite of trust.

I love to watch my cat Zeena and her brother Bo lying on their backs like rag dolls, legs outstretched, stomachs exposed, completely open and trusting. They have come a long way from being the fearful feral kittens that we discovered on our porch four years ago. Back then I would watch them through the screen door, but as soon as I opened the door they would bolt. I longed for them to trust me. I talked to them through the screen in a soft, reassuring voice, "You are safe little kitties. You can trust me." I like to imagine that it's much like my angels and guides, watching me from the other side of a screen, telling me, "You are safe, dear one. You are loved. Trust. Trust."

My cats are my gurus, showing me how to bare my belly, surrendering, trusting, fully open to life. Stephen Levine talks about softening the belly as a way of healing ourselves: "We store fear and disappointment, anger and guilt in our gut. Our belly has become fossilized with a long resistance to life and to loss. Each withdrawal, each attempt to numb our grief, turns the belly to stone. Have mercy on this pain you have carried for so long, the pain that sometimes makes you want to jump out of your body."

He advocates softening our belly by bringing loving attention to it. He says, "As we soften around the sensations and gradually move into them, they melt at the edge. It's not opposing the hardness but rather meeting it with soft mercy, knowing that we cannot let go of anything we do not accept."

I have begun talking to my belly the same way I talked to the fearful feral kitties on the other side of the screen, the same way I imagine my higher self is talking to me: "I love you. You can trust me. You can let go. You are safe. I will take good care of you." As a result, my belly softens, my heart opens, my throat relaxes, and my mind quiets. The belly is control central; once it is soft, my whole body softens and relaxes, and breath comes easily.

I've been listening for the voice of my higher self, talking to me through the screen. I recently had the thought that if I knew I was going to die soon, I would walk in nature every day. Instantly a voice came to me, saying, "Do it now." I am now walking in nature every day, breathing through my soft, trusting belly, listening to the sweet whispers of my higher self, "You are loved. You are safe."

Do you hear the voice of your higher self, talking to you through the screen door? What is it saying to you?

## 11

# FAMILY LEGACY
(May 6, 2009)

Last night I had a dream that I was at my grandmother Signe's house with my husband Tom. She wasn't home. Tom and I were in her bedroom, lying on her bed, talking. I was feeling scared that my grandmother would come home and find us on her bed; I was afraid she might think we had been "doing it".

Suddenly, I heard her enter the house, walking quickly down the hall towards us. Startled, we guiltily jumped out of bed. I tried to smooth the covers but they got caught on me and instead I pulled them off. Busted! She stood at the doorway looking at us. She was not smiling. I told her, "We weren't doing anything." I knew she wouldn't believe me. I felt a sense of shame, like I was bad and had done something wrong.

My grandmother Signe (long deceased) has been in my consciousness lately; I've been writing a story about her and her mother, my great-grandmother, Johanna. The story is focused mainly on Johanna. There is an intriguing family mystery involving her. She came to the United States in 1881 from Sweden, a pretty young girl in her mid twenties, and worked as head laundress at the Vanderbilt mansion in New York. She became pregnant out of wedlock and family rumor has it that the father was possibly one of the Vanderbilt sons. (This has never been confirmed.)

Johanna moved away and gave birth to the baby, my grandmother Signe. She lived in secrecy about who the father was. In those days there was a great stigma about having a child out of wedlock. I've been wondering lately, is there a legacy of shame in my family that got passed down either genetically or behaviorally or both? I know that my mother had a shame-based attitude. I have also felt the terrible weight of shame in my life; as a teenager I became deeply depressed and suicidal, feeling that I was bad, and that I would never be loved. Shame is more than the feeling that we've done something wrong; it's the feeling that we *are* something wrong.

As I'm exploring this, I'm wondering if an inherent imprint of shame around sexuality could have been one of the factors in my having uterine cancer? My mother also had uterine cancer. It is not unreasonable to think that blocked energy in a part of our body makes that part susceptible to disease.

Sometimes I imagine that I am helping to heal this ancestral legacy of shame. Maybe the work that my ancestors didn't finish, I can help finish, as if I'm in a relay race, carrying the baton forward. Carl Jung has written about this: "I feel very strongly that I am under the influence of things or questions which were left incomplete and unanswered by my parents and grandparents and more distant ancestors. It often seems as if there were an impersonal karma within a family, which is passed on from parents to children. It has always seemed to me that I had to answer questions which fate had posed to my forefathers, and which had not yet been answered, or as if I had to complete, or perhaps continue, things which previous ages had left unfinished."

I once awoke from a dream with these words resounding in my mind, "All you have to do in your whole life is to love yourself. That is all you have to do." The shame and deep depression that I've felt in my life have galvanized me over the years to focus on learning to love myself, every square inch of me, the inside and the outside, the upside and the downside. I feel like I have made great strides in that direction. In the past I often felt the impulse to hide myself, concealing my imagined ugliness. I now feel compelled to reveal myself, to be completely open, honest, transparent, and self-accepting.

My great-grandmother Johanna had tremendous strength and courage to sail to a foreign land, to have a child out of wedlock, and to keep and raise that child. I like to think that strength and courage is also part of our family heritage. Two psychics have told me that my grandfather Charles (Signe's husband) is nearby and is sending me love. It is comforting to think that I am being watched over. As I carry the baton forward, facing, revealing, and loving all of who I am, I imagine my ancestors cheering me on from the sidelines.

Do you have a family legacy? How is your amazing relay race going?

# 12

## MY 'TRUST' FUND
(May 10, 2009)

(Written Thursday, May 7)   I look out my window on this dark night and watch in frightened awe the wind-whipped Jesusita fire glowing in terrible beauty for 5 miles across the Santa Barbara mountains. My heart pounds as I see that a portion of it is racing towards us! There are urgent sounds of sirens, helicopters, planes, and a roaring wind; it sounds like war.

During the day the winds had died down, and the fire slept (after destroying 75 homes the night before); it seemed we were safe. But the sundowner winds awakened the fire with startling speed into a house-devouring monster that is now spreading out of control. We are on the outside edge of the evacuation zone and if the call for evacuation comes we are faced with the questions: "What do we take with us? What is important? What can we do without?"

I am adrenalized and frantically packing essentials. Then, Tom and I stop what we're doing and look at each other. Holding our gaze, he tells me, "Whatever happens, we will be fine." I take a deep breath; I know what he means. We know how to come fully into the moment, into the here and now, and be in that state of grace where everything works out. That is our "Trust" fund, which we have access to at any time. Even if we were living in a newspaper tent under the freeway, if we are in the moment, in that state of trust, we are safe.

During the course of this fire, flashes of awareness have

been coming to me that cancer is like a fire. My cancer is apparently "out", but my doctor said there is a medium risk of recurrence; there are possible embers that could be whipped into a raging fire again, a body devouring monster, spreading out of my control…like my imagination! Sometimes I am aware of a frantic energy in me, trying to make myself relax; afraid that stress, like the wind, could whip the embers of cancer back to monstrous life. Then I am reminded of my "trust" fund, and I take a deep breath, knowing that I will be fine no matter what happens.

It is now Sunday. Over the last three days the marines landed and saved Santa Barbara—the marine layer that is, blanketing us all in cool, moist protection. I am letting out a big sigh of relief. Tom and I went to a dance today where people gathered to commune and share our mutual experience of having been under siege and having survived. There were people at the dance whose homes had burned to the ground; they had come to dance their pain of loss and their joy of community and survival. Dancing can be an act of healing ourselves—animal's bodies naturally tremble once danger has passed, releasing the energy of the trauma. Dancing is a way to do the same.

I danced my body in rocking, shaking, releasing movements, like a saltshaker, releasing sweat and tears as my heart welled with compassion for those who had lost their homes. This spilled over into compassion for all of us who have had great losses in our lives: homes, breasts, uteruses, relationships. Dancing, shaking, releasing stress and deep sadness, moving through the wreckage and rising from the ashes, as passion comes, igniting flames of rebirth and celebration—such is the dance of life.

Fires are a natural part of life. They serve a beneficial purpose. The fires in our personal lives can do the same, but that depends on how we choose to look at things. Perhaps it is no coincidence that last week there was a Buddhist sand painting exhibit in town, which was exquisitely detailed and beautiful. Then they purposely destroyed it, demonstrating the transitory nature of material life and letting go of attachment to how things are.

It is freeing to learn how much we can let go of—whether it's a lost home, relationship, or uterus—we manage to rise from the ashes and recover our passion to recreate our lives. The human spirit has wings, like the phoenix, that carry us to new heights and new life. "Be as a bird perched on a frail branch that she feels bending beneath her, still she sings away all the same, knowing she has wings."-(Victor Hugo)

What is really important to you? What is it you would take with you if you had to suddenly leave your house? What do you want to take with you when you leave this life? I'm taking my "trust" fund!

## 13

## CULTIVATING LOVE
### (May 21, 2009)

What if you thought that you might only have a short time to live? What would you be doing with your life? Where would your focus be? Ever since my cancer diagnosis, I've been asking myself these questions. I saw my doctor a few weeks ago for a post hysterectomy check up and he told me that because there was a medium risk for my uterine cancer to recur somewhere else in my body, he recommended doing both chemo and radiation.

I am choosing to do neither of them. It doesn't make sense to me at this time to do something so debilitating to my immune system when we don't even know if there is any cancer left. What I am choosing to do instead is to continue with my strict diet, AND...to radiate myself on a daily basis with the healing energy of love! My soul lights up at the thought, saying, "Yes!"

Cultivating the energy of love in my life is the work I have been doing for years. It is what laid the groundwork for a wonderful, incredibly loving man to show up who matched that vibration (that would be my husband, the wondrous Tom). It is a law: if you build the energy of love, love will come. Now I have the motivation to turn up the volume on that.

Love has healing power. I'm not referring to romantic love; it is more powerful and permanent than that. Love is a state of connectedness, wholeness, union, and harmony with all that is. In the book *Healing with Love*, Dr. Leonard

Laskow writes, "Love stimulates healing by relating us to the natural order and harmony inherent in our cells, in our selves, and in universal consciousness. Healing through love is a process of becoming whole."

Even though I feel a strong intention to focus throughout my day on love, I know that inspiration wanes and, fears can take over; I tend to be a worrier. Fortunately, I am also a warrior. My spiritual warrior is very practical and has prompted me to implement daily practices that help plant me securely in the energy field of love. I want to share with you some of these practices.

1. LOVING SELF-TALK. I come into union with myself by loving my feelings as if they are my children, treating them like a mother would treat a beloved child. I bring loving attention to them, call them "honey" and "sweetheart", talking to them in an accepting way, and allowing them to express themselves. Once our feelings are fully seen, allowed and experienced, we expand into our full flowing aliveness.

2. THE WORD 'LOVE'. I lace my day with the word 'love'. Just saying or writing the word 'love' affects our cells. In Masaru Emoto's book, *The Hidden Messages in Water*, he writes how the effect of words on water molecules revealed that positive words like 'love' created harmonious patterns in water molecules, and negative words created disharmonious patterns. Since we are largely made up of water, it makes sense that the words we say to ourselves and each other have a powerful effect on us.

3. VISUAL REMINDERS OF LOVE. I put a picture of myself as a child where I can see it everyday. I look into that child's eyes, I see her beautiful soul, and say, "Hello sweet girl. I love you." My teenage niece told me recently that

she had been making some decisions that were emotionally hurtful to her. Then she saw a picture of herself as a little girl and she realized, "I'm hurting that little girl." That helped her to feel self-compassion, and she started making decisions that were more loving to herself.

4. ACTIVATE YOUR HEART CHAKRA.  HeartMath Institute has created a simple 3-step formula that stimulates the energy of love in your body: First, focus on your heart. Next, breathe through your heart. Finally, generate the feeling of love in your heart by imagining someone or something you love. You can also imagine bathing your heart in green light, the color of the heart chakra. I have an Emwave device from HeartMath that gives bio-feedback and helps me know when I am in that state (the light turns green when I'm in 'love', and red when I am not).

5. NATURE LOVER. I take daily, love-generating walks, communing and harmonizing with nature. On a recent walk I was inspired to write this poem, celebrating our 'love affair':

NATURE IS MY LOVER

*The sun warmly kisses my face.*
*The ground holds me in earthy embrace.*
*The wind playfully tussles my hair.*
*The gift of flowers scents the air.*
*My lover gives me lots of space.*
*And let's me move at my own pace.*
*Though some would say there's no one there,*
*I deeply feel this love affair.*

Abraham Lincoln said, "It's not the years in our life that counts, it's the life in our years." Ultimately, it's the love in our moments that truly counts. I think that is what we take with us when we die, how much we have opened our heart, our cells, and our being to love. Even if I were to die a year from now, if I am filled with love, I will have accomplished a huge thing, I will have done one of the most important things that my soul came here to do.

If you thought you might have a short time to live, what would you be focusing on? What generates the energy of love in you?

## 14

# AN 'EMERGE AND SEE' SITUATION
(June 3, 2009)

We are all on a hero's journey of awakening. We have been entranced by the stories we tell ourselves about our lives, ourselves and each other. Convinced that our stories are true, we are spellbound to only see and experience our life from that limited perspective. It is a great triumph on our hero's journey to awaken from our trances and discover that we are the authors of our life stories.

One of my prominent story lines used to be "Poor Janet". I was a captive of, and captivated by, that story. It was a part of my identity. I received attention and validation for being "Poor Janet". I remember once when I was about seven, I was at a birthday party and I wasn't winning any of the games or prizes. I then played a game of my own…I sulked in my best "poor me" demeanor, and the mother hosting the party took the cue and gave me a prize! Though our stories confine us, they also define us and reward us in some way. That's why we stick to our stories and they stick to us.

For many years, when it came to relationships, I felt the lingering imprint of my "Poor Janet" story, the main theme being, "Nobody wants me. I will always be alone." There's a Snoopy cartoon in which Lucy is lamenting, "Nobody loves me." Snoopy is standing next to her, lips puckered and says, "I love you, sweety." She doesn't even see him. She says, "No one cares about me." He says, "I do, I care about you." She continues to be oblivious to his presence and says, "Probably no one will ever love me." Snoopy finally gives up and says, "You're probably right, sweety." Like Lucy, I wasn't able to see love even if it was there because it didn't fit my story.

Eventually the pain and boredom of my story awakened me from my trance and I could finally see how I was perpetuating it. I was then ready to create a new story. A breakthrough moment came during the first week I met Tom, almost exactly ten years ago. He was at my house and we were massaging each other's feet and I was in oxytocin heaven, and thought, "I'd like to have this in my life, long term." A Bonnie Rait song began playing and I was singing along with it, "I can't make you love me if you don't." That song activated the neural pathways of my sad old story that read, "I will always be alone. He won't want me. I can't have this."

I caught myself slipping into the bittersweet melancholy of that story, and I stopped and thought, "Wait a minute... why can't I have this? It's just habit programming. I'm just as lovable as the next person. I can have this!" In that moment I had a clear awareness that this was MY movie; I am the star, director, casting agent, and writer of my movie. I can chose to do a conscious rewrite!

I decided to change my story. I once read that Barbara Streisand said early in her career, "I have decided to be beautiful." I decided to be loved! I backed that decision up with actions that eventually helped to completely revise my story line. Now, ten years later, I'm continuing to share regular oxytocin moments with my husband Tom.

I find that old neural pathways and story lines can be re-stimulated in times of stress. This past year, "Poor Janet" (and the fear and sadness that fuel her) has been tugging at me, saying, "First my appendix burst, then cancer, then a hysterectomy, then fires blazed through the Santa Barbara mountains. What a horrible year!" Or, as Queen Elizabeth once said, it's been an "Annus Horribilis".

This year has challenged my sense of safety. It has confronted me with the fact that anything can happen. Anything! I really don't have control. A hot sundowner wind can suddenly appear and whip up a fire that burns scars into the beautiful mountains and peoples lives; cancer can scar and take away parts of my body, or even my life. Fear asks, "What if my story turns out to be a tragedy after all?"

Fortunately I have a larger part of me now that keeps me from being seduced into that old storyline; I know that our stories are shaped by how we choose to interpret what happens. Holocaust survivor Victor Frankl said, "The last of one's freedoms is to choose one's attitude in any given circumstance." My choice now is to bring compassion and loving presence to WHATEVER is happening. Compassion is a great awakener and unifier. Bringing compassion and loving presence to "Poor Janet" (or any other trance state) whenever she shows up, comforts and calms her and integrates her into the whole of me.

From this vantage point I can see that the events of my life this year have created an *'emerge and see'* situation; I am *emerging* to a higher perspective and *seeing* clearly what I want to do in my life: to align with my souls purpose, to be fully present here and now, and to reinforce the awareness that love is the answer—loving what is, loving all my feelings about what is, loving myself for not loving what is. It's all about love. That's my story. It's a Love Story!

What's your story? Is it a tragedy? A comedy? A love story? A story of despair? A story of triumph? Are you in an "emerge and see" situation? Once we awaken from our trances and see that we are the authors of our stories, we can create a new story. Here's to living Happily Awake Ever After!

# 15

## ALL LIFE IS AN EXPERIMENT
(June 10, 2009)

Ralph Waldo Emerson wrote, "Do not be too timid and squeamish about your actions—all life is an experiment." That quote keeps coming to my mind lately as I am faced with changes in my life. I take a deep breath whenever I think of it: "All life is an experiment; therefore," I tell myself, "relax, accept change, be willing to take risks and make mistakes for the sake of living your fullest life."

When I was a young girl in grade school a teacher once wrote on my report card, "Janet will one day learn that it's a waste of time to worry so much about making a mistake." It was about the same time that I was taking sailing lessons at the Mystic Seaport. The other kids were sailing all around me on the Mystic River, tilting, capsizing, having great sailing adventures and playing with the wind, while I just sat there, stalled, afraid, playing it safe, unable and unwilling to catch the wind.

The winds of change have been huffing and puffing around me this past year; a ruptured appendix, cancer, and a wind-whipped voracious fire in our mountains have reminded me of the impermanence of this earth life. I feel my soul urging me to fully live my life while I am alive, to let go of the safety, security, and stagnancy of the known and to follow my dream and concentrate on writing.

My mind says cynically, "Yeah, right, follow your dream to the poor house!" My mind is like an anchor, resisting the wind, trying to keep me moored in the familiar. But the winds of change are blowing my mind, rocking my boat, and exciting my soul, who is joyously singing "Anchors aweigh!"

Someone recently sent me the inspiring story of Phoebe Snetsinger, a 50-year-old woman who was diagnosed with cancer and given a year to live. She decided to forgo treatment and use some inheritance money that she'd received to travel around the world as a birder. She ended up living 18 more years (she died in a van accident) during which time she became legendary in the birder world for having seen and recorded more birds than anyone else in the world. She threw caution to the wind and followed her bliss and it led her to a rich, rewarding life.

Sometimes when our world is blown apart, we are freed from the safety and inertia of the familiar, and are challenged to make changes, take risks, and follow our hearts desire. However, we don't need our world to be upended in order to do that. For the last two years my husband Tom has been committed to concentrating his time and resources on developing and marketing his ingenious right-brain math system (he's Mister Numbers on youtube with over 500,000 views). He's excited and tail-wagging happy every day to be living his dream and making a difference in people's lives. He inspires me to do the same, as does this excerpt from "The Invitation" by Oriah Mountain Dreamer:

*It doesn't interest me what you do for a living*
*I want to know what you ache for*
*and if you dare to dream of meeting your heart's longing.*
*It doesn't interest me how old you are*
*I want to know if you will risk looking like a fool*
*for love*
*for your dreams*
*for the adventure of being alive.*

My soul is urging me to take a leap of faith, to open my heart like a parachute and leap into the unknown, trusting the direction the wind is blowing me. Maybe some of you are feeling the urge now to take a leap of faith and follow your heart's desire. If so, "Do not be too timid and squeamish about your actions—all life is an experiment."

## 16

## CAN YOU HEAR ME NOW?
(July 3, 2009)

I've been immersing myself this week in news about Michael Jackson's death, planting myself like a vegetable in front of the television and the computer, reading about and relating to his anxiety and insomnia, and the drugs he used to relieve them. My 3-month checkup at the Cancer Center is due, and I've been feeling anxious, unable to sleep, and have been "drugging" myself with television and the Michael Jackson drama. The immersion distracts and disconnects me from my fear, but it also disconnects me from my spirit. The voice of my higher self, growing ever fainter in the distance, is saying, "Move your body. Take a walk." I move my body over to the couch, pick up the remote control and search for more MJ news.

I can see how being stuck in the contracted energy of fear has kept me from doing my daily disciplines of dancing and walking, actions which help me connect with my spirit. It's like when we lose connection on our cell phone; in order to reestablish connection we need to keep moving to another position, asking, "Can you hear me now?" until the reception is clear. I have lost clear connection with my spirit, but my spirit hasn't moved out of range of reception…I have, by numbing my fear with hours of escapist drama.

I'm aware that whenever I feel occasional twinges of pain, fear is activated and my worried mind asks, "What is that? Is it cancer?" Fear is like a barking dog, barking at the slightest noise. The barking is now waking me up, reminding me that I have moved out of range of my higher voice, reminding me that it's time to take my inner barking dog for a walk in nature and get reconnected to my spirit... taking my God for a walk. When I change my position and move my body, I get unstuck and can then hear the voice of my higher self, reminding me, "You are safe. You are so much more than a body, so much vaster than your fear." That helps put the fear into perspective—it's just a little bitty scared dog nipping at my heels.

As I nervously sat on the exam table waiting for the doctor to come in, I literally shook my body like a dog shakes water from its fur. Shaking helps release the grip of fear. I acknowledged to myself, "I feel scared." That always invites a big spacious breath. Then I affirmed, "I am so much more than a body." I imagined the vastness of my spirit inside and all around me, and I calmed down. When the doctor examined me and said, "You're fine. I'll see you in 3 months," I was tail-waggin' happy!

Deepak Chopra said that when his friend Michael Jackson danced on stage, "It was there that he was no longer a person in emotional distress, but instead someone dancing in the world of the spirits." Dancing, shimmying, shaking, moving our bodies helps loosen the grip of fear and allows us to reconnect with our spirit.

Fear is a great motivator; it is designed to be compelling in order to get us to take survival action in the form of fight or flight or freeze...OR, to take 'thrival' action by facing into the fear, feeling it fully, and therefore freeing ourselves from it. I have felt compelled this week to face my fear, feel it, and free my body to move into a place where the reception is strong and clear. My higher self asks, "Can you hear me now?" "Yes, I can hear you now."

What is your current response to fear? How do you connect with your spirit? Is the reception clear? Is it time for some movin' and groovin' to the tune of your higher self?

# 17

## M.I.R.A.C.L.E.
(July 9, 2009)

My brother Norm has been living with a brain aneurysm for years—and I mean LIVING! Nine years ago he was wracked with an excruciating headache. The doctors discovered that it was from a leaking aneurysm, and rushed him into surgery. After a 7-hour brain surgery, they determined that his aneurysm was inoperable. When he realized that he could die any day, he chose to LIVE every day. He followed his bliss and bought a sailboat and sailed to the Caribbean where he is having wonderful adventures in paradise. He stopped thinking about the aneurysm and lived as if it was gone. A few weeks ago he had an MRI, which showed that the aneurysm has completely calcified and there is no longer a threat of it rupturing!

He sees this as a miracle. What I see is that he had a powerful intention to live as if he were whole and healed. The seed of intention that is well tended and nourished can flower into coincidences, synchronicities, and miracles that heal the body, boggle the mind, and lift the spirit. I've created an acronym for the word miracle:

*My Intention Radiates Apparently Coincidental Luminous Events*

When these "coincidental" luminous events happen to me and the people in my life, it reminds me that there's more going on than meets the eye; there is an unseen energy that responds to our deepest and most focused desires. Einstein said, "Coincidences are God's way of remaining anonymous." For me, they are God's way of saying, "You are not alone."

Prayer is another form of intention that reveals our connection with the powerful forces of the Universe. In my early twenties I was feeling deeply depressed and asked for a sign from God that life was worth living. Just then there was a sound of movement in the room. I looked in the direction of the sound and saw that a candle in a candleholder on the wall had fallen to one side, pointing to the calligraphed poster next to it that read: GET THY SHIT TOGETHER. I smiled to myself and thought, "Is that you God?" The next day as I was writing about it in my journal it happened again! It excited me and made me want to stick around, to live, play and explore in this magical energy field of life.

Another time, several years ago, I was having another "dark night of the soul", feeling deep despair and praying for guidance. As I was crying and journaling about it, a card that was displayed on the bookshelf beside me fell to the floor. I picked it up and it had a rainbow heart on the cover with the words, "You are so loved."

I love how when we're open to it just the right words, experiences, and people that we need fall into our life. It is  perfect timing that my brother has recently shared his healing miracle with me; it inspires me to let go of thoughts of cancer (knowing that I have made all the healthy life changes I could) and continue to focus on seeing myself whole, healed, and connected to the miraculous forces of the Universe. That's the intention I want to radiate.

I believe that the deepest intention of our soul is to be vibrantly present, whole and alive. Adversities can be valuable and necessary stimulants in bringing about that intention, resulting in the miracle of our full participation and appreciation of life and living our wildest dreams.

Do you have an intention that is bringing forth miracles in your life? Is there adversity in your life that is serving as "miracle grow" to help you flower into more vibrant aliveness and living your dream?

## 18

# GO WHERE THE LOVE IS
(July 16, 2009)

On Sunday Tom and I drove up the coast to pick some peaches at the beautiful El Capitan Ranch, where groves and gardens adorn the hillside overlooking the ocean. Everything on the land was thriving: there were huge, fragrant, happy looking roses of every color, a datura tree resplendent in angel trumpets, succulent peaches, and oil-rich avocados.

The woman who owns and works the land told us how she nourished everything that grew there with a special ingredient...LOVE. It was clear that she is in a heartfelt love relationship with the land, the trees, the plants, and the flowers. She told us that she talks and listens to them, and they guide her in how to care for them. That love gave birth to the sweetest, juiciest peaches I have ever eaten. (Love tastes good!).

I believe that when we are in love with what we do, we are guided, and wonderful things come from that. I have been in a love relationship for over 25 years with my muse, creating crafts to sell at the Sunday Santa Barbara Arts and Crafts Show. I named my company after my muse, A-Muse Ink. Over the years this love has spawned many "children". One of the first of these children was a little pig, which came into being this way: I said to my muse, "I need something that will make people say, 'That's too cute, I have to have it.'" I wanted it to be something that was easy and inexpensive to make.

Then a vision came to me of a pig wearing sunglasses

lying on a rock, "bacon in the sun". That day, in magical synchronicity, just the right materials and equipment to easily make the pig presented themselves. After a period of labor I gave birth to my Bacon in the Sun line of pig magnets and flying pigs. Through the years I have often heard people say about them, "That's too cute, I have to have it". Those little guys helped me bring home the bacon!

I have loved being in relationship with my crafty muse and with the Arts and Crafts Show all these years. However, relationships can eventually become stagnant, the joy is gone and we fall out of love. I was feeling that with the show— it had lost its sparkle for me. It became more a drudgery of labor than a joy of birth. I was feeling labor pains for something new to be born. Then, several months ago, I was diagnosed with uterine cancer.

I don't know if the cancer was born of that stagnancy, which in turn gave birth to the impetus to do something new that excites my soul and stirs my juices. What I do know is that is the result. The fatigue I was feeling because of the cancer and subsequent hysterectomy, caused me to quit the show. In the meantime, I have been developing a relationship with a new love, my writing muse. We have intimate conversations, and I listen and receive guidance. This love is birthing the "muse" letters I've been writing to chronicle my journey.

I feel excited about this relationship with my writing muse. This new love is juicy and sweet, like the peaches at El Capitan Ranch. While I was going through the experience of cancer, I felt more captivated by the joy of writing than the fear of cancer. It is a loving partnership that I nurture by taking walks in nature, and eating healthy foods that keep me clear-headed and better able to connect with that higher part of myself.

Like any good relationship, the more I talk to it, the more it responds; and the more I listen, the more I hear. Sometimes my mind is blank, I don't know what to write and my muse assures me, "Relax, just listen, it will come." And it does.

My mind sometimes has doubts about fully committing to writing. Yet my higher self is urging me to take the leap into the unknown and compelling me to "Go where the love is and trust you will be guided." And so I am.

Are you in a love relationship with where you are and what you're doing in your life? Are you feeling urges to go where the love is? Trust that when you follow the love, all that you need will come to you.

# 19

## MENTAL AIKIDO
July 23, 2009

Albert Einstein said, "I think the most important question facing humanity is, 'Is the Universe a friendly place?'" One of the reasons that this question is so important is that scientific research has verified that how we perceive the Universe affects our stress level, which in turn affects us at a cellular level, greatly impacting our health and quality of life. In other words, believing in an unfriendly Universe can literally damage our cells and make us sick, not to mention miserable.

Most of our beliefs are formed at a very early age and become deeply ingrained. By the time I was 19, I felt trapped in an unfriendly Universe, locked in the cage of my hardwired beliefs. I began searching for a key that would free me from that cage. One of the things I did was read the book, *The Power of Positive Thinking.* I found that learning to think more positively did help; however, I also found that there was more to it than that. In fact, when we try to force positive thoughts that we don't really believe, the critical part of our brain becomes activated and resistant. Our critical mind scoffs, "Nice try Pollyana, but you can't fool me."

I eventually learned that the best way to change a belief and shift a feeling is to first come into union with it. In the spirit of Aikido, a Japanese marshal art in which you blend with the energy of the opponent, (Aikido literally means "way of adapting the spirit"), you can be with beliefs and feelings in that same way by aligning with them, listening to them, being present and accepting them as they are. Then— here's the key to changing it—give it a twist upwards by adding onto it a true and positive suggestion that shifts it to a whole other place. I call this Mental Aikido. To anchor this concept, just imagine…what does A Key Do? It aligns with what is there and then you give it a twist upwards and it opens the door to a whole new state of being.

For example, when I'm sitting at the dentist office in the electric chair—I mean dental chair—I have often felt terrified. I actually twitch and tremble sometimes and have even been known to cry on occasion. I feel like a big weeny! If I tell myself, "Just relax, you're safe, this will be over soon," it doesn't help me. Trying to push away my fear is like trying to push a basketball down in water. It just doesn't work.

What I've learned to do instead is to align with the fear and flow with the energy of it by saying to myself, "This is scary isn't it? Someone is poking at your gums and teeth with a sharp instrument. I totally understand your feeling scared. It's okay to feel scared. Let yourself feel it." Then something amazing happens…I feel seen and heard, and my breath softens and my body starts to relax a bit.

That creates an opening where I can give an upward twist by introducing a true and positive suggestion, telling myself, "I think you are courageous for coming here and taking care of your teeth, even though you're so afraid. You have done a great job finding a caring and highly competent dentist who knows what he's doing and is gentle with you. You are taking such good care of yourself. I'm proud of you." I begin to relax even more, trusting myself, seeing myself as a courageous winner, instead of a wimpy weener.

I've been using this Mental Aikido over the past several months with my experience of having uterine cancer. My fear of cancer was one of the bogeymen hiding in the shadows of my Universe. I have come face to face with this bogeyman, accepting that it is what is, allowing and fully feeling the feelings that have come up. Then I turn the key upward, opening my mind to a friendly Universe by focusing on the great gifts that are coming from this experience, such as seeing the courage I didn't know I had, feeling appreciation for the gift of life, and making a commitment to live my dream and do what I feel passionate about. Through the magic of Mental Aikido, the bogeyman that was cancer has been transformed into an ally in my spiritual growth, and my Universe is transformed into a friendly place.

What is your experience of the Universe? Is it a friendly place? Do you have beliefs about your world that are keeping you from feeling safe and happy and living your fullest life? I highly recommend using Mental Aikido as a key to transforming your perception and experience of the Universe. It is a powerful tool that can help us answer Einstein's question in the affirmative: "Yes, the Universe IS a friendly place."

**20**

## FEAR IS A RECURRING VISITOR
(August 5, 2009)

I've been waking up in the morning for the last few days with some nasty bug bites on my body. Not many, four so far, but they are big, red and painful. Last night I was afraid to fall asleep, thinking that IT, whatever it is, would come out in the dark of night when I'm sleeping and vulnerable and bite me again! I'm thinking it may be one of those big, thick, gnarly-looking black spiders. I imagine it cunningly waiting for me to fall asleep so it can crawl onto my body and sink its fangs into me like a mini vampire. Is it any wonder that I was wide awake until 3 in the morning!?

I believe that life is a mirror, and that whatever shows up in my life is reflecting some part of me. I asked myself what this is trying to tell me. The thought came to me…something is 'eating' at me. What is it? I sat with that question for a few seconds and then I realized what it is…I am afraid that cancer may still be lurking in my life, waiting to take a bite out of me, or it may already be gnawing away in the dark unknown of my internal body. Cancer is something that literally eats at us; it ate my uterus!

I had decided to try and stop dwelling on it, like my brother who stopped thinking about his brain aneurysm, which then eventually calcified. But there is a very fine line between not dwelling on something and repressing it. How do you know when you have let something go or are just whistling in the dark? For me that's easy—sitting on my feelings is very much like accidentally sitting on my felines—they very quickly bite me in the butt and I am forced to face them.

As I am now facing my fears, I realize once again that the worst part of cancer for me is the anxiety about it. That is what I'm resisting; that is what was eating at me like a spider in the black night. What I resist persists, in one form or another.

Now that I've brought my creepy crawly thoughts into the light of awareness, it's time to do some Mental Aikido with them, coming into alignment with them, telling myself, "I know that you're scared. It's okay to feel scared. Let yourself feel it. It is natural to feel scared about cancer. It's something we don't have much control over. That is scary." Deeper breaths come as I allow the fear, and I am ready for the up-twist. "It's true that cancer might reoccur, AND, right now you are fine, right now you are healthy and strong and right now is all there is." I take a big breath into open space.

I am accepting that fear is a recurring visitor to my life, a teacher that is helping me strengthen my faith muscles, build my 'trust' fund, and create a belief in a friendly universe. It is also teaching me to feel compassion for myself and for others who suffer with fear and anxiety. I want to hug us all in love and strength and say, "Yes, I know what that feels like. I understand. Just know that we are so much bigger than our fear. We are so much vaster than a body. We are so loved and watched over." Fully feeling my fear always leads to feeling the loving presence of my Big Soul Self.

Is there something in your life that is trying to get your attention, something that is 'bugging' you, some disowned part of you that is eating at you? Shine the light of awareness on it, and invite it to the party—there's plenty of space for all of God's critters that show up.

THE GUEST HOUSE by Rumi

*This being human is a guest house.*

*Every morning a new arrival.*

*A joy, a depression, a meanness,*

*Some momentary awareness comes*

*As an unexpected visitor.*

*Welcome and entertain them all!*

*Even if they're a crowd of sorrows,*

*Who violently sweep your house*

*Empty of its furniture,*

*Still, treat each guest honorably.*

*He may be clearing you out*

*For some new delight.*

**21**

# PRECIOUS CARGO
(August 18, 2009)

Do you ever get the feeling that you're not alone—the feeling that you're being watched over and guided? I love that feeling! I just read a book about spirit guides, which said that we all have guides who connect with us throughout the day, whispering to us, making suggestions, nudging us. After I read the book, I felt compelled to connect with my guide. I got out my Osho Zen Tarot deck, shuffled it thoroughly, closed my eyes, asked, "Please speak to me," and randomly picked the card titled "Guidance"!

It read, "The angelic figure with rainbow-colored wings on this card represents the guide that each of us carries within. In following the inner guide you will feel more whole, more integrated, as if you are moving outwards from the very center of your being. If you go with it, this beam of light will carry you exactly where you need to go."

I smiled, feeling reassured...I am not alone. Whatever you choose to call it—higher self, angels, guides, God—I know that there is some higher energy that travels with us through life; we are carrying a precious cargo. When I'm aware of this precious cargo, I hold myself differently; my posture is more uplifted, reaching upward, yet grounded at the same time, like a flower. When I'm not aware of this higher energy, my posture has a tendency to bend forward, as if folding myself up.

I first became aware of my bent posture in the 1966 movie, *The Group*. I was sixteen at the time it was being filmed, and I was an extra playing a student on the campus of Vassar College in the opening scenes of the movie. Director Sidney Lumet instructed me and another girl to walk past opposite sides of the camera from behind, coming together in front of the camera and walking off into the distance, merging with other students on campus.

When I saw the movie I was surprised to see that this shot was the very first scene in the movie. I was also surprised to see myself, blonde braid down my back and wearing a long green skirt appropriate for the 1933 setting, shlumping along like a vertical turtle. It appeared as if I was tucking my head slightly forward and down. If posture could speak, mine would have said, "I'm not sure I want to be here in this movie, on this planet, in this body known as Janet."

Over the years, I have committed to being in my body, and to following the directions of my higher self. I have been directed to do yoga, be Rolfed, and get numerous chiropractic adjustments. Yet my body, like memory foam, still tends to fall back into its comfortable, familiar shlumping posture, and the beliefs and attitudes that accompany that posture. It is an ongoing learning process, revealing to me that when I change my posture my attitude changes, and when I change my attitude my posture changes. My body and my guides are my learning buddies, letting me know when I have slipped into old unconscious attitudes and holding patterns.

I have witnessed that in addition to 'turtling' inward, my body sometimes has a tendency of hurtling forward, in an urgent hurry to get somewhere other than here. One day a few years ago I was walking in a parking lot, with lots on my mind, when BAM!...I tripped and slammed down to the ground with great velocity, my head smashing into a bumper of a parked car on the way down. I sat on the ground stunned, with little birdies and stars circling my battered head. I wondered, "How did that happen?!"

I realized that I hadn't been present in my body, I wasn't

over my feet, I was in my head and my head was ahead of myself. I was ungrounded and the universe obligingly grounded me! I was asleep and the fall woke me up!

I have a deep desire to wake up, to be present, to remember who I really am and why I'm really here. When I forget, I am reminded...at first by whispers...but when I don't listen to the whispers, they become shouts. That fall was a shout, just as cancer has been a shout, saying, "COME INTO YOUR BODY! COMMIT TO BEING HERE! SAVOR THIS MOMENT! TREASURE WHO YOU ARE! HONOR YOUR DEEPEST DREAMS! WAKE UP!"

I am now wide awake! My feet kiss the ground with every step. Whenever I notice myself turtling or hurtling, I recommit to being fully Here in my body, and make micro movements, lifting my head and ribcage, dropping my shoulders down, creating a posture and attitude that says, "I am carrying precious cargo," affirming, "I choose to be here, in this body, in this life, in my movie called Waking Up."

I went for a walk the other day, and on the walk I imagined that my guide was appreciating me, showering me with love and acknowledgement for my commitment to being in my body, for staying in touch with higher energy, for honoring my body and soul by exercising and eating healthy foods that help me be clear and able to hear the voice of my higher self. As I tune into that voice I realize what it most wants me to know is that not only am I carrying precious cargo, I AM precious cargo, as are we all.

If your posture could talk, what would it say? What are the things your guide loves and appreciates about you? What is your guide directing you to do? Listen to the whispers. We are not alone; we are being watched and guided and loved unconditionally. What a feeling!

## 22

# THERE'S GOLD IN THEM THAR ILLS!
### (September 9, 2009)

I read something remarkable recently that moved me to tears. Eighteen-year-old Shawn Hornbeck, who was abducted by a predator at age eleven and held in captivity for over 4 years, wanted to share some of his insights about the experience with Jaycee Dugard, who was also abducted at age eleven and was recently found after 18 years in captivity.

He said: "I had a lot of built-up anger afterwards, which is normal. Going to therapy really helped me get everything in order. One of the things that really helped me is that we talked about how I could better myself from what happened to me, how could I use all those terrible, awful experiences I had, to grow and mature. I know it sounds crazy, but those experiences have made me a better person."

Wow! After all the horrors that he'd endured, this young man turned his victim's journey into a hero's journey by finding gold in his experience, finding the gift in his wound, and sharing this gift with others. He also freed himself from the captivity of his anger and bitterness. That is the ultimate freedom! And it is no small feat.

I know what it's like to be a captive of resentment. It has been an ongoing teacher of mine. For years I was addicted to 'stewing', simmering in a soup opera of resentment, feeling victimized, wronged, and ripped off. Anyone who has ever been trapped in resentment knows what a powerful, addictive force it is. Hanging on to feeling wronged becomes more important than anything, more important than freedom from it, more important than love.

I vividly remember one day when I was about eighteen years old driving to work at the New London Submarine Base. I was stuck in traffic and stuck in a stew about my life, singing along with great, tearful emotion to The Young Rascals song playing on the radio, *People Gotta Be Free*:

*All the world over so easy to see.*
*People everywhere just wanna be free.*
*Listen, please listen,*
*That's the way it should be.*
*There's peace in the valley,*
*People got to be free.*

I felt a deep longing to be FREE from the captivity of negativity and anger. About that time in my life I began reading about how our thoughts and attitudes create our reality. The truth of that strongly resonated with me. I could see that it was my attitude that was creating my unhappiness. Nobody was MAKING me angry...*I* was responding with anger, and then dwelling on it, making myself stew, and creating a negative attitude that rendered me a shit magnet, drawing to me more things to be resentful about. I realized that my resentment was far more destructive that anything anyone could ever do to me. I was only hurting myself. I set out on a lifelong quest to free myself from the confines of my negative attitude.

On this quest I eventually learned to become a 'miner': I discovered how to mine gold from my anger by seeing what is MINE, seeing my part in things, seeing how I was contributing to my own misery, seeing that I can choose to hang on to anger or let it go. I can choose to be a bitter person, or a better person because of my experiences. I can choose to dwell in the hell of The Heartbreak Hotel, or dwell in love. I can choose captivity or freedom. And I can choose to mine gold from any situation...even cancer.

I must admit there are times when I feel bummed out, and wonder, "Why me?" It would be easy to slide down the slippery slope of resentment. But I'm choosing to use some of the keys to freedom that I've found along the way to help me through this cancer experience. When I notice myself feeling wronged and starting to spiral down into that sticky, stuck, stewing place, I do the following:

**I witness myself** – I observe the physical feelings of resentment, such as a tightening of my body, shallow breath, eyes narrowed, lips pursed. When I become aware of the contractive prison of my body enclosing me, and realize that I am doing that to myself, I take some deep breaths and begin to shift into a more expanded place.

**I accept that it is what it is** – I take a deep breath... accepting...there's nothing I can do about it...it happened... it is what is.

**I allow and align with the feeling** – I tell myself, "Yes, this sucks. I understand how you would feel upset. Let yourself feel it fully." My hard stance begins to melt, allowing me to feel the sadness that lies underneath the anger.

**I generate loving kindness towards myself** – I talk to myself with compassion, like I'm talking to a wounded child, verbally hugging myself. "I'm sorry this happened. I know this is hard for you. I'm here for you. I love you."

**Finally, I mine gold from the experience** – I learn from it and own what is mine; and then, I see how it has made me a better person, a stronger person, a more empowered person.

All this results in FREEDOM, with the added bonus of some gold nuggets in my pockets to share with others. There's gold in them thar ills and there's plenty for everyone! Just think, if Shawn Hornbeck can find the gold in his experience, then anyone can.

Have you ever been held captive by your resentment? What are ways you have freed yourself from that captivity? What is the gold that you mined from the experience?

## 23

# FROM WORRIER TO WARRIOR
(October 12, 2009)

Are you a worrier? The good news is, if you are someone who tends to worry, you possess two very special powers: the power of VIVID IMAGINATION, and the power of PERSISTENT FOCUS. People who are really good at worrying, like I am, are actually able to visualize and feel the thing they fear as if it were real; in addition, they have the ability to tenaciously focus on it. Those are super powers! The trick is to harness those powers and use them for expansion and growth (instead of contraction and stuckness). That's when the worrier metamorphs into the warrior.

Worry can be insidious. I believe that our thoughts and beliefs create our reality. That belief sometimes leads me to worry that my worry will create what I'm worrying about! I am worrying about worrying! If what I focus on grows, did my worry grow cancer? I urgently think, "Must stop worrying. Must think positive." But that is just another form of worrying.

Since worry seems to be a given for me, I have a choice to either use it to suffer or to grow. I don't like suffering, therefore, worry has been a compelling force in my personal growth. It is a burr under my saddle, a spur in my side; I am learning to harness it and take it for a ride, like a bucking bronco, riding out of the tight pen into an expansive field.

I want to share 5 ways that help me use the power of Vivid Imagination and Persistent Focus to transform my worrier self into my warrior self:

1. The first way is to imagine the worrier within as a child who feels small and powerless. Imagine putting that child into your heart, and speaking to the child affectionately, holding, comforting and loving the child. In the act of doing this, you become your compassionate, loving, Big Soul Self, which is who you truly are, and your little worrier self is put into perspective.

2. The second way is to use worry as a catalyst for prayer. People who worry are motivated to pray. Studies of prayer show that what makes it most effective is imagining and feeling the energy of what it is we desire, feeling as if it is already so. Native American rainmakers say that they don't pray FOR rain, they pray rain; they imagine it, they feel it. When my husband Tom first came to California he walked along the ocean shore longing to see dolphins, but none were showing up. His yearning contained the energy of lack, as if he were saying, "I want it but I can't have it." He recognized this, and shifted into feeling joy about the dolphins that he knew were there in the ocean, and he sent them warm feelings of appreciation. Before you could say "leaping dolphins" they appeared!

3. A third way is to imagine that Right Now is all there is. Worry is usually about a regretted past or an imagined future. You can use worry as a reminder to come into the present moment and be here one breath at a time, one step at time. My brother lived on his sailboat off the coast of Saint Croix and a few years ago Hurricane Omar crashed head on into the island and sank my brother's boat. He lost everything. He felt devastated and worried. A friend let him stay on his boat for awhile. My brother told himself to just take baby steps. He said to himself, "All I got to do is get up; all I got to do is get myself to shore in the dingy; all I got to do is take baby steps, one after another." A year later, he was a very happy

man. He learned that he had more friends than he ever knew he had because people generously reached out to him and helped him get back on his feet. Now he is living on his new sailboat that is even better than the one that was destroyed. What a difference one step at a time makes!

4. Fourth, imagine that your fear and worry are just frozen fun. Fritz Perls said, "Fear is excitement without the breath." Add breath to worry and you free up that energy, turning it into fun and excitement. I'll give you an example: I'm always nervous before giving a speech, but I've decided to breathe and call my nervousness excitement, and now I feel a lot better about giving speeches. I sing to myself, "I'm so excited. I just can't hide it. I'm about to lose control and I think I like it!"

5. Finally, people who worry tend to be sensitive. Sensitivity helps us feel things more deeply. Just imagine that though our sensitive thin skin leaves us less protected from pain, it allows us to be more connected to our spirit. What a blessing that is! I wrote this poem about this a number of years ago:

BRONCO RIDE

*You were born into a skin of vibrant sensitivity*
*so that you might better feel the magical nuances*
*that play through life.*
*Your challenge, brave one, is to use*
*the pain that penetrates that silken thin skin,*
*harness it like a bronco,*
*ride it where it might go,*
*trusting the grace of your being*
*and the direction of your flow.*

*Hang onto that bronco*
*with all the courage and spirit that is yours*
*and you will eventually see your landscape*
*change into one of such magnificence*
*that you will be glad for the ride*
*and remember why you came.*

*The sun is always shining above the clouds.*
*You will find your way back to the light*
*where treasures await you,*
*where you will remember*
*that you are the treasure,*
*you are the light.*

*So wrap your arms tight*
*around that bucking bronco.*
*Life is worth the ride.*

Is there something in your life that you're worried about? What are some creative ways that you can use the super powers of imagination and focus to transform your worrier into a warrior?

# 24

## THIS IS IT!
(January 1, 2010)

This is it—the end of a decade! This is it—the beginning of a new year! Most importantly, this is it—the eternal NOW! In the book "Wherever You Go There You Are", Jon Kabat-Zinn suggests that we say the words "This is it" throughout the day, reminding ourselves that right now is IT!

"This Is It" is also the name of Michael Jackson's farewell tour (and movie), a name that proved to be prophetic for him. I sometimes think that when world-famous figures such as Michael die at a young age, it is a parting gift to us all on a soul level, a wake up call that reminds us that This Is It! Be fully here and alive while you are here and alive, because you are not going to be here and alive forever!

My experience with cancer this year was a dynamic 'This Is It' reminder. It catapulted me into the here and now, helping me to appreciate and value this moment, cherish this life, and transform my "someday" dreams into "today is the day, now is the time." I always said that someday I would write and I am finally doing the writing I've always wanted to do.

Santa Barbara acupuncturist Bernard Unterman told me about a woman with stage 4 lung cancer whose doctors had told her there was no treatment that would help her and that she should check into hospice. She went to him instead. He asked her what brought her joy and she said "Nothing." Until she remembered that she once enjoyed doing art, but then her life got too busy. In addition to acupuncture, he prescribed that she begin doing art again, which she did. Within 5 weeks she burgeoned into a vibrant, vital woman and her cancer was gone! Growth happens one way or another.

When adversities happen we can either buckle under them...or buck up, using them as impetus to take a stand, commit to life and live it fully. Kenny Loggins sings passionately about this in his song This Is It. In an interview in *American Songwriter* magazine in December 1987 he talks about his inspiration for the song: "I had a fight with my dad when he was going into the hospital because he gave me the feeling that he was ready to check out." That inspired the lyrics: "You make the choice of how it goes...For once in your life, here's your miracle. Stand up and fight. This is it!" We make the choice of how it goes—we can choose to be here fully and to live our dream, or not.

When fear is dogging me, nipping at my heels, and I'm worried about dire possibilities, I take a deep breath and say, "This is it. This moment right now is all there is." I am taking a stand, making the choice to be here, fully embracing this glorious life one moment at a time. Mike Dooley in his Notes from the Universe wrote recently: "When driving down the road of life, rarely do you know how good you have it, until you see it in the rear-view mirror. Which is not to suggest that you should look back now, but to remind you that where you are today is more awesome and amazing than you probably realize."

This past year I have learned to treasure my life, recognizing the miracle that it is, realizing that our time here is limited, and recommitting to fully live while I am alive. This is not a dress rehearsal—This is it!

I'm wishing for all of you a passionate love affair with this eternal now moment. May you do what brings you the most joyful growth in life.

## 25

## FACING THE UNFACEABLE
(February 27, 2010)

I just came face to face with a massive issue I've been avoiding, and I have my butt to thank for it. Lately I've been spending a lot of time messing around on the computer, watching TV, and eating. I recently did something I haven't done since my diagnosis and removal of cancer a year ago. I have been faithfully avoiding sugar (it feeds cancer) and dairy, but the other day I walked to the Fresco bakery (voted best desserts in Santa Barbara!) and I got a big slice of berry pie with homemade whipped cream. I was proud of myself for bringing it home and sharing half of it with my husband Tom.

Two days later I went back and got another yummy dessert (a caramelized banana marzipan flakey pastry), but this time I didn't share it with Tom. I didn't even tell him about it. It was a sweet, secret treat that I hoarded and hid and ate all by myself.

Big fat red flag! There have been other red flags that something was up, or held down, something I didn't want to face. A few weeks ago I had a severe ear infection and blockage in my left ear with pain radiating into my neck and face. I couldn't hear out of that ear and I felt unbalanced. In addition, for several weeks my butt has been unrelentingly aching with painful hemorrhoids, the grapes of wrath! So I asked myself, "Your ear aches and your rear aches, what's up with that?"

I'm taking antibiotics for my ear and it's better. But the

pain in my butt is not going away. My rear aches everyday, like a tiger's got ME by the tail. The persistent pain scares me, with the thought that cancer is always a possibility. I tried to reassure myself that everyone gets hemorrhoids (it's said that's why Napoleon rode side saddle!) But then a lady from the community garden told me she had hemorrhoids and it turned out to be anal cancer. Oh My God, my worst fear! I googled anal cancer and hemorrhoids and my fear mushroomed.

Fear has taken over! I am out of balance; I've lost touch with my spirit. In trying to avoid this fear by distracting myself with TV, food, and the computer, I have also separated myself from my spirit. I have been spirited away by the addictive distractions that fill my day.

My ear aches and rear aches are fear aches. I've been tightly clenched, trying to push fear away, avoid it, sit on it. But once again I am reminded that when I try to sit on my feelings, they bite me in the butt! And it's very painful! I am now willing to come face to face with my ear, rear, and fear aches.

Laying in the spaciousness of Tom's arms, I let myself go into the depths of my fear and sadness about cancer. Even though it was removed, I have a creeping fear that it will return. I face into the surprising awareness that a part of me would rather die than to go through more cancer, pain, hospitals, expense, needles, knives, blood, and fear!

I cried and released and unwound my pain, and then…I became aware of Tom holding me, and I felt the sweet space he was providing me, and I suddenly remembered how I used to cry and feel this same deep despair years ago when I felt so alone in the world. Now here I was with Tom.

My eyes opened wide, taking in this present moment where I was held and loved. I awakened to this wonderful moment and I smiled, happy to be alive, feeling my feelings fully, in the spaciousness of the here and now with this beautiful man.

I can see that my butt has been aching to communicate with me, trying to tell me, "Get off your butt. Take walks in nature. Reconnect with your spirit." My hemorrhoids feel better when I'm moving, walking and breathing fully, and they hurt when I'm sitting around distracting myself with mindless activities.

I am hereby committing to reconnect with my spirit, to meditate, to walk in nature, to call my doctor and check it out, to face my fear, to breathe fully and recommit to life.
Later today Tom and I are going for a walk in nature. We're going back to the Botanic Garden where I haven't been since the Jesusita Fire ravaged it several months ago. I haven't wanted to see it's marred beauty—I didn't want to face it. Today I am willing to face everything.

How about you…is there something you haven't wanted to face? Have you been distracting yourself? Is the universe probing you with aches and pains and discomforts to wake you up? Nestle into the spacious embrace of the present moment and let it all hang out. You will feel so much better.

## 26

# MY WORST FEAR
(March 13, 2010)


Wednesday I was stunned to hear from my oncologist the words that I most feared, "Your cancer has returned." A tumor the size of a small lemon is growing between my vagina and rectum, causing the pain that I mistook for hemorrhoids. I am surfing tsunamis of sadness, fear, and disbelief, as well as a spiritual uprising. I feel galvanized into the present moment as I watch myself alternate between fight, flight, and light.

My oncologist said that I have about a 50% chance of survival with chemo and radiation. I told him I was considering doing alternative treatments instead. He folded his arms and told me that I then would have a zero percent chance.

I just finished reading Suzanne Somers book "Knockout" which has interviews with alternative doctors who are having success with their treatments. She builds a case against radiation and chemo, saying they do more harm than good, pointing out that many conventional doctors don't have the big picture, they have only been trained to see cutting, burning or poisoning as a way to deal with cancer.

I am aware that I have a distrust and fear of doctors from early childhood traumas. I saw the plates of sugar cookies in the Cancer Center waiting room, and my distrust intensified—
—don't they know that sugar feeds cancer?

As I explore my relationship with doctors and hospitals, I see that I hold a feeling of being victimized and wronged by them, and a belief that they make things worse. There were lots of balls dropped in my cancer diagnosis that delayed treatment by a year. I also have a belief that cutting into the cancer for a biopsy makes it spread. And then there's the thievery of hospitals price gouging and charging exorbitant fees. Why is a CT scan $4000?!

I feel mad, sad and scared about doctors and hospitals. The memory just came to me of getting my tonsils out when I was five-years old...I was having a bad dream, apparently making moaning noises, and the nurse was angrily slapping me, telling me to shut up. I want to go back and slap that nurse!

This unresolved fear and anger has been making me want to build a case for alternative and against conventional treatment. I can see that the Knockout book's prejudice against chemo and radiation, saying that it doesn't work, is just like my oncologist saying that alternative treatments don't work. It is black and white thinking. It is a dueling duality. Alternative treatments do work for some, and chemo and radiation does work for some as well.

I've been demonizing chemo and radiation to bolster my case for doing alternative treatment. I thought my resolve was coming from a conscious, higher place, yet I see that it was my ego disguised as my higher self, putting the 'con' in conscious. It was my fear-based, victimized ego righteously choosing alternative treatments over that 'evil, greedy, life debilitating' conventional medical model. I need to clear this childhood trauma and prejudice so that I can make a decision from the big picture, rather than the little case that my ego has built.

What I know for sure is that I have a very strong spirit. I look at Tom and am reminded that I can create miracles. For most of my life I had an emotional blockage in my heart, I didn't love myself, and didn't believe anyone could ever love me. Then I decided, "I want to have love in my life. I am willing to do whatever it takes." And I did it! I cleared the blockage in my heart and learned to love myself and let love in—that's when this miracle called Tom came into my life.

This cancer represents to me the blockage of fear, distrust, and resentment that is within me. My work is to face, embrace and heal this blockage. I am very clear that if I do check out, I want to check out without any emotional baggage. I think that's why I'm here. I know that's what I feel passionate about. My soul is saying, "You can do this!"

Once again, I'm choosing to think of cancer as a 'growth' opportunity. I'm all about growth and I intend to continue to go for the most conscious growth I can get out of this growth!

Is there a growth opportunity in your life that you're seeing as a problem? Much light and love to you and to me as we grow to our highest potential.

## 27

# HAND IN HAND WITH MY BIG SOUL SELF
(March 20, 2010)

On Thursday I consulted with an alternative doctor, Dr. Issels in Santa Barbara, about my recurring uterine cancer. I told him that 3 months ago my gynecologist didn't feel any mass inside me, and now I have a lemon-sized tumor. He was alarmed that it had grown so large in such a short time and said I needed to do something immediately. Even though he favors an alternative approach, he said this is like a train and it needs to be stopped. He suggested that chemo and radiation might stop the train, at least temporarily; and then do the alternative afterwards. PANIC!

I'd been straddling the fence between alternative and conventional, but this pushed me over. Toxic poisoning be damned...I've got a train roaring up my butt! Tom got me an appointment the next day to get a PET CT scan (he found a relatively low-priced one in Ventura). That is the first step that needs to happen before we can proceed.

This week I also saw Pamala Oslie, a trusted Santa Barbara psychic, and she told me she saw the little girl in me who was scared and unhappy with life and didn't want to be here and wanted to go Home. I'm well aware of her, I have always had one foot out the door. As a child the world seemed an unfriendly place with a cold, critical mother and a distant father. Even though I am so happy now in my life with Tom, and despite all the work I've done on this, it appears that that part of me still exists.

Pamala said I needed to convince little Janny that life

is good now and we want to be here…or else little Janny is going to go Home and take me with her! She's a powerful little thing! On my bedroom wall I put a picture of myself when I was two years old with my round baby face and wispy blonde hair. Next to it I put a picture of Tom when he was two. Little Tommy is looking over at little Janny with a twinkle in his eyes and a sweet smile on his face. Janny looks like she's been crying, she looks mad, sad, and scared. I look at her and say, "Look who's next to you. He's really nice and fun. He really loves you a lot. He's taking good care of you. He wants you to stay and be with him."

Yesterday while driving with Tom to get the PET CT scan, Janny was nervous, terrified of clinics and hospitals. She would rather die than go to those scary, pain-inflicting places. My Big Soul Self took little Janny by the hand; we are going through this together. In the waiting room I held her in my lap and kept talking to her. "I'm here with you, I'm taking good care of you. I won't let anyone hurt you. You can trust me. It's okay to let yourself feel scared, or mad, or sad. I'm not afraid of your feelings. You can feel anything you want."

The nurse who was performing the scan was nice; her name was Janet like mine, and her middle name was Lee, also like mine. (Turns out that our fathers had a thing for actress Janet Leigh). As she was about to inject the radioactive glucose into a vein in my hand, little Janny clenched in fear. I talked to her, "This is a nice lady, she's here to help us." Feeling a slight prick, I said to my scared self, "There, that wasn't too bad, was it? We can do this."

I imagine that the just-injected solution that is coursing through my body is friendly, is here to help me. I know that how I think and feel about something affects me more than the thing itself. If I imagine it as toxic and fear it, then that thought will make it more toxic. If I imagine it as healing and helpful, it will be received by my body in that way.

I was then led into a warm, small, dimly lit room and laid down on a comfortable cushy chair and told to relax for 45 minutes, not moving as the liquid potion moved through my body. I held little Janny in my lap, imagining that healing light was filling us and surrounding us. "This is nice, isn't it? Peaceful." This was a time to really talk to her. Thinking of sweet Tom in the waiting room I said, "Look who we're with, a wonderful man. We're having so much fun with him and he loves us just the way we are. We're learning so much together. We have fabulous friends, and live in a beautiful place. Life is really good now. We've found our way to a safe and happy place."

As I'm lying there a fart escapes me, and little Janny clenches in a fear and shame reflex. What if the nurse comes in and smells it!? Hearing my mother say "Ish." I learned to feel embarrassed and ashamed about this part of my body and have always been *down*tight. I say to Janny, "That was so good that you let that out! Good girl." I smiled, imagining angels applauding. Little Janny started to relax on my lap, breathing softly…then farted again. The angels cheered and applauded wildly.

Janet Lee comes in and leads me to the CT scan where I lay down and, with arms over my head, I surrender and am slowly rolled into this box. I close my eyes, afraid of tight spaces; I'm in a bit of panic. I open my eyes and see the top is just inches away. It feels like a coffin. (Note to self: Cremation). Breathing slowly, I become my big soul self, holding this scared child, loving her, talking to her gently and sprinkling us with healing, shimmering white light. I actually relax and almost nod off in this enveloping box.

After a half hour, Janet Lee rolls me out and sends me on my way, telling me, "Don't go near little children for the rest of the day, because you're radioactive." I smile to myself, walking out embracing my little girl, glowing as I reconnect with my beloved Tom in the waiting room. This was a healing experience for me.

I meet with my oncologist on Wednesday and he will tell me the results of the scan. Has it spread to other parts of my body? I'm scared. I don't know if I'm going to do chemo or radiation or alternative treatment. I do know that I will be immersed in my big soul self, embracing and loving little Janny, loving my fear, loving this life, and letting in all the love that is coming my way.

Is there a part of you that could use a hug right now? Let's breathe into our Big Soul Self and embrace all our wounded little ones, as we love, hug, and heal ourselves into wholeness.

## 28

# FREEING THE GENIE FROM THE BOTTLE
(March 26, 2010)

I've heard that the experience of death feels like a genie being released from the bottle. Life can feel like that too, when we free ourselves from the tight confines of our fears and programming. I am opting for the life version of releasing my genie, uncorking the big energy of my bottled-up life force.

I have put myself on a healing program that includes dancing, bouncing, shimmying, and shaking every morning to move lymph through my body, reduce stress, oxygenate myself and free up my expanded energy field...and I am doing it in my yard outside! I am boldly going where I dared not go before!

In the past my fears have kept me from dancing outside, fears that the neighbors might judge me, embarrassed to reveal my white dimpled arms and legs, afraid that being barefoot outside might cut my feet on something, scared that sunlight causes cancer. But now, barefoot, bare arms and legs, I am shaking and shimmying my pelvis like Elvis for all the neighbors to see. All my fears are coming to light, coming to dance in the light.

As I was dancing I noticed that at times my shaking, bouncing, and shimmying had a frantic element in it. I wasn't moving in harmony with my fear, I was moving in disharmony, trying to get away from it. That shook loose a big learning for me—I see that so much of what I've done to protect myself from the big bad scary world, doing 'all the right things', has been fear-based.

I've been trying to control my world by carefully avoiding toxins and dangers. I've been anal retentively trying to maneuver my ducks in a row and keep them there. But all my efforts to get my ducks in a row just quacks them up! The fears underneath those efforts to protect myself have proven to be more toxic that what I've been trying to protect myself from. Fear has become a cork in my bottle, and, literally, in my bottom, in the form of a tumor. It is time to unclench! To pop my cork! To face and release the energy of my fear and anger and full aliveness.

A friend told me of someone she knows who loves to swim in the ocean but is afraid of sharks. He decided to imagine himself swimming into the jaws of the shark, right into the belly of the beast. He met his fear head on and the fear subsided. I am meeting my worst fear head on, I am facing the beast in my belly, cancer, and seeing that it's just a frightened, pissed off little girl, curled up in a ball, in a fist, in a fetal position.

I say to her, "Come sweetheart, let's blow this popstand! Let's explode into our full aliveness! You have a right to be here, to be fully here, with all your piss and vinegar, all the colors of your being. Let yourself be big and bold and alive! The universe awaits us with open arms!"

Clearing this blockage, healing this little girl, and uncorking my aliveness has become my passion and my mission. I have kept my two cats, Bo and Zeena, captive inside, afraid to release them into the dangerous world of coyotes and fleas and cars and other cats, afraid that I might lose them. They look out the window longing to explore the rich, scary, exciting world outside. In the spirit of liberation, I am freeing my kitties! I am opening the door and releasing them to this great adventure of life! I'm excited for them. I'm excited for me.

This is the great challenge of my soul, to face my worst

fear, to face death, to face life. My brother has just set out to sail around the world, stirring his juices, rousing his soul, facing his fears. His adventure sounds more fun. But nothing is as important and exciting to me as meeting this big soul challenge.

Of course, I have waves of deep sadness, fear and anger, but I'm intent on riding those waves to solid ground where I remember who I really am—I am a soul on a great adventure, here to face and free my blockages, to uncork my full aliveness.

Are there places in you where your aliveness has been corked? I invite you to unclench, uncork, free that energy, and let your magnificent, big, bold genie self out of the bottle!

**29**

# THE MIRACLE-PRONE ZONE
(April 3, 2010)

Because of my health crisis I am experiencing accelerated growth...emotionally, spiritually, and, unfortunately, in my tumor. My little bundle of growth (opportunity) is literally a pressing issue, and despite my onslaught of alternative healing modalities, the tumor is aggressive and requiring immediate and much stronger action.

I saw a radiologist last week and he wants to begin treatment right away. Tom and I pressed him to give us a ballpark percentage of the cure rate and he reluctantly said it was about 20%. That's not good. He said chemo would probably add another 20% chance. Ouch. (Surgery is not an option because of its size and difficult location).

My mind took those figures in and deduced, "I'm toast. This is a crapshoot. It's a long shot. Why go through all that misery and have it not even work?" My breath was sucked out of me and I became engulfed in a crushing anxiety of such magnitude that I hoped to be zapped by lightening or a heart attack right then and there. Panic screamed, "Get me out of here! Put me out of my misery!"

This was my mind run amuck, which can be a very dangerous thing. The mind, seeing dire possibilities, concentrates on that outcome to the exclusion of any other outcome, and through the power of that focus brings about that outcome. A voice within urgently said, "You are in danger girl! Get yo butt to the miracle-prone zone!"

That is the place beyond mind, it is meta-mind; it is beyond physical, it is metaphysical. It is a magical place where anything is possible, where miracles happen. It is that faith-fueled state of grace where everything we need flows to us easefully, where a flourish of 'coincidences' occur and things turn out better than our limited minds could ever imagine.

How do I get to that magical realm? How do I become miracle prone? The old song comes to mind, "It's so high, we can't get over it, it's so low, we can't get under it, it's so wide, we can't go around it, we gotta go through the door." Going through the door means opening to facing and feeling my feelings fully, letting the river of tears flow and flow and flow. Once spent, I take a big breath of acceptance, "Here I am, this is what's happening. Now…here…this."

Feeling and breathing is ventilating the situation, bringing oxygen and light to it, which eventually allows a stillness where healing love and energy can fill and surround me. Being porous to that energy carries me to the spacious field of the miracle-prone zone—while being in the energy of "poor us" keeps me closed off from that powerful healing energy field. Therefore, moment to moment, I have a choice to become expanded and porous or stay contracted and stuck in "poor us."

In my research I've found that cancer is anaerobic and thrives in low oxygen. Fear and anxiety exist in shallow breath and create a fertile environment for cancer to grow. The energy of faith and trust stimulate slow, deep, easy breaths, creating an atmosphere for healing and miracles.

A friend of mine recently showed me her impression of the Arabian stallions she saw recently. They are very spirited, with their heads held high, tossing their manes grandly and strutting their magnificent stuff with great panache. When I am aware of myself moving in a way that is trudging along, in an energy of "poor, poor pitiful me," like an old grey mare, I remember my friend's impression and I change my stance and I start to prance and dance like an Arabian stallion, tossing my mane, and feeling my supreme value. By doing that I change my biology, I stimulate life-enhancing energies within me, and I project that out to others and they reflect that back to me. I prance my way right out of the "poor me, moan and groan zone" and into the miracle-prone zone.

Another powerful way to become miracle prone is to come purely, wholly, completely into this…eternal…now… moment. Time magically expands in the eternal now and we are freed from the confines of time. Tom and I have been meeting eyes, drinking in each other and the moment, slowly breathing in, breathing out. Now. Now. Now. All time is Now. In this spacious present there is plenty of time. Abundant time. Right now I am here. Right now I am alive. Right now I am breathing fully. Right now life is beautiful.

I have been anchoring my awareness in the realm of miracles by making note of the 'coincidences' that have come from being in the flow. Like the woman administering my PET CT Scan who was named Janet Lee, just like me. She had a healing, loving presence that helped de-traumatize my experience of medical care. I also consulted with an elderly colonics healer named Alice, my mother's name. My mother installed in me the 'ISH' issue, shaming my elimination functions. This Alice, who even looked a little like my mother, was someone who celebrated and encouraged elimination, helping me to heal my ISHues.

I am focusing on the miracles that have happened in the last year and a half, reminding my skeptical mind of the unlimited possibilities that have come my way. My appendix burst and was necrotic and gangrenous, and I survived! That is a miracle! Houdini died of a burst appendix—that great escape artist could not escape that fate. But I did! And miraculously, most of my medical bills were handled by a financial assistance program (I have no insurance). The same thing happened for my hysterectomy a few months after that. I call that 'mira-cal' health insurance, and feel very blessed.

I have been immersing myself in the Seth books, which remind me that right NOW is the point of power; anything we have set in motion with our thoughts and beliefs can be changed in this NOW point of power. I have discovered to my surprise that there are Seth books I wasn't previously aware of called *The Magical Approach* and also *The Way Toward Health*, both are about how to enter the metaphysical field of unlimited healing possibilities. I'm reading those books now, and in them Seth is advising Jane Roberts (who channeled Seth) on how to deal with her life-threatening health problems. I have my handwritten letter from Jane Roberts on my bed stand, reminding me of our vast powers and possibilities.

I also look at my cat Zeena and am reminded of the death sentence she received from the vet not too long ago… yet Zeena lives! A miracle! I loved her back to life.

Then of course, there is the wondrous Tom…the greatest miracle of my life. I was hardwired to live my life alone, but through the power of intention and getting myself into the miracle-prone zone, Tom came into my life and we continue to thrive in a beautiful, loving, learning, fun, playful, spiritual partnership that just keeps getting better and better.

I believe in miracles. Miracles do happen. That is the energy field I want to continue cultivating and living in. I know that I am healing the emotional blockage this tumor represents. Whether my body goes along with this emotional healing, I don't know. That's out of my hands. I will do all that I can do and rest in the spacious field of the miracle-prone zone. I would consider the healing of my emotional blockages in this lifetime a major miracle. I believe that chemo and radiation may be the next adventure, the next growth opportunity to heal my fears and beliefs, and, hopefully, it will yield the next miracle.

Are you ready for a miracle in your life? Then get yo butt to the miracle-prone zone and be ready for surprises!

**30**

# RADIANTLY ALIVE!
(April 16, 2010)

Yesterday I began my first radiation treatment. I awoke at 4 this morning all aglow, abuzz, bright-eyed, bushy-tailed, and radiantly alive! I have committed to a course of treatment that involves six weeks of radiation, 5 days a week, 20 minutes each session. I will also be receiving chemo once a week, a low dose to help the radiation work better. I may even get to keep my hair, though I bought a really cool wig just in case. I have leapt fully into this adventure, 100% committed to it, finally. Even though I haven't been given great odds by the doctors, I'm an odd person, so that adds to my odds, right?

The last few weeks I have been on a wild ride emotionally, bouncing around between decisions like, should I do alternative treatment, conventional, some of both? At times, when facing these life and death decisions, I have felt crushed by anxiety, and in that state I've wished that this life was over, finished, kaput. I have careened from a desolate sense of being abandoned, to being in an exhilarated state of wild abandon, letting go, letting it all hang out. Facing and accepting death can be very liberating!

In that spirit of wild abandon, Tom and I have freed our housebound, indoor kitties, Zeena and Bo, into the world. Watching them tentatively put first one paw, then the other in slow motion over the door threshold to a whole new world was like watching my children take their first steps. They are freed from a mother's fear to explore the wild and wonderful world outside. My sweet kitties are now carnivorous hunters, hunting prey (instead of each other) and proudly bringing their terrified prizes home to their terrified mama. There is a lizard hiding under the refrigerator right now!

As part of this journey, Tom and I have unclenched around our money issues. At first, when this all began, there was the question for me: "Your money or your life?" Hmm, I'm thinking, I'm thinking. And for Tom, "Your money or your wife?" But, like Zeena and Bo, we have been freed, sprung from the tight confines of our money fears. We are now willing to completely let go of our money—opening our hands and our hearts like parachutes, we leap, trusting we will land securely in our 'trust' fund. Geronimo!

During these last few weeks I have been confronted with an old persona of mine, a cynical voice that keeps piping in. A nurse asked for a list of the supplements and herbs I take, which are numerous. She said, "Wow, you take a lot." "Yeah, a lot of good it did me," I said bitterly. I hear my 80-year-old neighbor hacking next door from years of smoking cigarettes, and my cynical one sneers, "That cig-sucking old lady is probably going to outlive me!"

Cynny (my cynical one) feels like a victim. The world is against her. She is doomed and damned pissed off about it. From this cynical one's perspective, chemo and radiation are just a further assault. "Yeah, right, I go through all that agony and torture and I probably die anyway." The chemo doctor told me that my cancer is in a bad place (pelvic area) and will be very painful as it grows, and even if the treatment gets it to move to another place, that would be a good thing because any place else is better than where it is. Cynny thought, "Oh great. Can this nightmare get any worse!?"

I used to live in that negative attitude—now I just visit it. It is a good yardstick for how far I've come. When Cynny pipes in, I play with her, exaggerate her. She likes to wallow in the moan and groan zone, so I make the moaning and groaning even moanier and groanier. Just how bitter can I let myself be? I play with bitter until I feel better.

I see so clearly…that is one of the big healings that needs to happen…that bitter attitude, and the fear and sadness that lie beneath it. This is an opportunity for me to heal that old wound, to befriend this experience by reframing the chemo as 'chemo sabe', seeing it as a friend instead of a fiend, imagining it as a healing elixir intent upon helping me.

While receiving my first radiation treatment yesterday, I visualized shimmering angels directing the beam of light right to the tumor, and protecting the surrounding tissue. When the treatment was done I was told that the machine they are using is the best in the world, the state of the art Novalis, a cyber knife designed to do minimal damage to healthy tissue, and maximal targeting of the tumor. The radiation therapist said, "Somebody likes you."

Then there is Tom, whose presence in my life reminds me that miracles are possible. He also reminds me, "This is all about soul growth. It's all good. We're right where we're supposed to be." He is the perfect partner for me on this journey, helping me to remember that this is happening for my higher good, it is about learning, healing my soul, and my emotions. This is the big healing, the big show, this is it! In this awareness, I feel excited about the opportunity for some big-time soul growth.

I recently read about someone who referred to himself as 'cancer enlightened' instead of 'cancer survivor.' I like that. I am becoming cancer enlightened, radiating from this experience, shining the healing light on all that is ready to be healed.

Is there something in your life that is ready to be healed, to be radiated, to be played with, to be loved? Heal-elujah!

## 31

# YOU ARE SO LOVED
### (April 24, 2010)

I've heard that some people sail through chemotherapy. I was hoping I would be one of those fortunate sailors. Alas, I am a seasick sailor. I started chemo last Monday and it has shivered me timbers and left me a bit woozy and bluesy.

I have felt myself shlumping like an old gray mare this week, suffering with a queasy stomach and no appetite. I'm trying to remember my chemo sabe attitude of last week, but instead, I'm feeling chemo sobby—as in boo hoo, this sucks! I don't want to get stuck in the energy of that old gray (night)mare. But I also don't want to be "false positive".

I went to a doctor appointment yesterday, and while in the waiting room I eavesdropped on a concerned father who was talking on his cell phone to his obviously distraught daughter:

"I want you to know I love you very much," he said to her. "I love all of you, just the way you are, the good and the not so good, every single thing about you I love. It's okay to cry. Tears are good. Things grow in a wet environment. Let yourself cry all that you want. It's helping you grow. I am so proud of you. I know this is hard for you, and you're doing wonderful. Just put one foot in front of the other, one step at time, that's all you have to do. I love you so very much."

Tears came to my eyes. He was like an angel father from heaven, talking to her so tenderly, showing how supremely precious she was to him, saying all the things a suffering daughter craves to hear, allowing her to be right where she was. I imagined that he was my angel father speaking to me so lovingly and tenderly. Angels are all around us.

I am reminded of the time several years ago, when I was feeling down about myself and I prayed for help. At that moment a card that was displayed on the shelf beside me floated to the floor. I picked it up and it read: "You are so loved." That was such a powerful reminder to me that I am not alone, I am being watched over, I am loved. A few weeks ago I taped that card to my mirror so I can see it everyday and be reminded of that.

I am now being an angel to myself, talking to myself in a loving way, like that father talked to his precious daughter. "I love you very much. You are being so brave. You are facing your worst fears. Just take one step at a time, one foot in front of the other. It's okay to cry. Let it out. You are doing great. I am so proud of you. Know how very loved you are."

I opened the Pema Chodron book I've been reading, *The Places that Scare You,* to this angel-sent quote: "The 'secret' of life that we are all looking for is just this: to develop the power and the courage to return to that which we have spent a lifetime hiding from, to rest in the bodily experience of the present moment—even if it is a feeling of being humiliated, of failing, of abandonment, of unfairness."-(Charlotte Joko Beck)

Then laughing angels flipped the book open to this quote, "In the garden of gentle sanity, may you be bombarded by coconuts of wakefulness." -(Chogyan Trungpa Rinpoche). I love that! I am being bombarded by coconuts of wakefulness! I tell myself, "Wake up and love yourself right where you are. Breathe into this moment, allowing, accepting, embracing all that is happening, crying when you need to, and laughing too."

The funny thing is, as I do this, I begin to breathe and relax, and the queasy feeling becomes a more easy feeling. I can see that my resistance to what is happening created more discomfort and queasiness than the chemo itself. Resistance is a powerful force—and so is acceptance.

Is there something in your life that you've been resisting? Is there something that's been rocking your boat? Be an angel, and love love love yourself just as you are, right where you are.

# 32

## FINDING A NATURAL HIGH
(May 9, 2010)

I've been feeling like an immigrant from olden times, sailing on a ship across the ocean, once inspired by a dream of a new life, but unable to feel that inspiration because I'm too darn seasick! I want to touch solid ground. I want to feel good again. I want to enjoy food. I want to remember the dream.

Today I have landed on an island of solid ground, and reconnected with inspiration and my dream of health, and I ate delicious, nutritious whole-wheat waffles for breakfast! Usually by the weekend, the further away from chemo I get, the better I begin to feel. But chemo rolls around again tomorrow, every Monday, another wave, as I resume my ocean voyage.

Last week I had high hopes for a new anti-nausea pill that I was trying out. I felt a little bit naughty…it's called Marinol, a synthetic form of marijuana containing THC. It is supposed to improve appetite and reduce nausea (and I was also secretly hoping for a nice mellow high). I'd only smoked marijuana about 3 times in my life, in my twenties, and I didn't like it; I felt paranoid. Now we were to meet again, legally. I wondered how we would get along.

As I took the pill last Tuesday, I was writing this newsletter. Within minutes I found myself reading the same sentence over and over again, unable to get a grip on it… the Marinol had kicked in! My eyes started spinning like little pinwheels and I quickly shut them. Crap! I was trapped in this dizzy spinning wheel for the duration of the dose. I held perfectly still, eyes clamped shut for 2 to 3 hours, with creative ideas flickering in and out like fireflies, then gone forever. I was dizzy for days afterward—so much for my 'high' hopes for this drug.

As I rest on this island of solid ground today, I am taking deep, slow breaths, evoking a natural high, the remembrance and feeling that I am right where I'm supposed to be—simply being still and quiet and resting in this spacious place. I have been reading my Bartholomew book by Mary Margaret Moore, which reminded me that, "We have misidentified ourselves as the clouds, when in fact we are the vast sky." I am focusing on identifying myself as the sky, and peacefully watching the clouds go by.

Last Monday, as I sat in my 3rd chemotherapy session, I closed my eyes and became the sky, witnessing my inner clouds. What I saw was a lifelong pervasive story of mine that was clouding my perception, coming up to be healed. When I first enter the chemo room I search for the perfect chair where I can plant myself for the 3-hour intravenous treatment. I want a nice, private area. I don't want to chat with people, I want to be quiet and read and meditate.

The 'clouds' gather as I imagine the nurses watching me and judging me as a difficult, fussy, unsociable patient. Then I witness myself trying to counter their imagined bad opinion of me, trying to be 'good', trying not to be a 'problem'—in other words, not asking for things I need and want, like a pillow or a blanket or water. I get mad at myself for being such a wuss. Why shouldn't I ask for what I want? That's what these nurses are here for, to help, right?

I begin to judge the nurses. Nobody really looks at me or offers to help, except when the buzzer goes off and they come over and press some buttons and dash away. I watch them chat and joke with friendlier patients, and I conclude, "Oh, I AM the problem." Now I am in high school comparing myself to the outgoing, cool kids.

Thoughts come like: "Why can't they meet me where I am? Why can't they ask how I'm feeling?" As I witness my thoughts, I know that I am projecting my story onto the nurses. I'm amused at myself as I watch the 'clouds' drift by, and I become more and more the observing sky. Or, as Pema Chodron wrote, "You are the sky. Everything else—it's just the weather."

In this witnessing place I realize that I am meeting myself right where I am—I don't need the nurses to do that. I am celebrating my quiet nature, my need for privacy and time to reflect and being still. I imagine like-minded friends meeting me in this spacious place. I imagine my husband Tom and all the people who love me just as I am.

I open my eyes and high school and uncaring nurses have disappeared. There are only efficient nurses waiting for me to ask for what I want. I ask and they happily give it to me. These clouds were just wisps of past programming, the old core belief that my very nature is a "problem" for those around me. In the clearness of this vast blue sky, I appreciate that some very fine healing happened at this chemotherapy session.

Tomorrow is Monday, another chemo day. My goal is to anchor myself in the feeling that I am the vast sky, even in the midst of gathering clouds and stormy seas and seasickness. Finding peace within the storm is a challenge that inspires me. It is a dream worth remembering.

What are ways that you re-inspire yourself and remember your dreams in the midst of life's cloudy skies and stormy seas?

# 33

## JUST SHOW UP
(May 15, 2010)

This morning I was in the waiting room of the Cottage Hospital Lab to get a blood test. In the next room I heard the frantic, pleading screams of a little girl named Emmy, "Nooo, nooo, nooooo!" The nurse was trying to draw her blood but Emmy was having none of it. She protested over and over again, screaming, crying, railing against her present reality, trying to outrun it, resist it, fight it.

Several of us who were in the waiting room witnessing this human drama gave each other knowing smiles. How many of us have had, or still have, a child inside of us screaming those same words, "Nooo! I don't want this! Get me out of here!"

Her mother and the nurse were wrangling with her, telling her, "Emmy, just sit still, don't be scared, it will be over soon." I wanted to tell them, "Move toward the fear. Tell her you know how scared she is. Tell her it's okay to be scared. Meet her where she is."

I had a wonderful private phone counseling session yesterday with Mary-Margaret Moore, who channeled the Bartholomew books in the 80's and 90's, books that bring me more comfort and feelings of expansiveness than any other books I've ever read. With heartfelt compassion she counseled me to move toward my fears and pain and not resist them, to simply rest in them for a while, to be present with what's present, to stop efforting, stop trying to be elsewhere, even in a "higher" place, because, to paraphrase

Bartholomew, "You are already there, and once you effort you have lost that place."

In the session I got in touch with a painful belief that I have done something wrong, I've screwed up, I wasn't relaxed enough to keep the cancer monster away; my fears and tension drew it to me. As much as I have felt empowered by the belief that my thoughts and feelings create my reality, there is a downside to that belief; there's a blaming and shaming of what I have created. Mary-Margaret asked me to question that belief, to ask myself, is that true? Did I create it? Can I know that for sure?

The only thing I can know for sure is that cancer is here. Chemo and radiation are here. Nausea is here. I am here. When I stop resisting it and wanting it to be different, then I land on it—I show up and come into harmony with this reality. Breathing and resting in what's happening, no matter what it is, is the portal to the spacious NOW. Kicking and screaming and resisting, like little Emmy, is what creates most of the suffering, just as arguing with and resisting Emmy's fear only compounded it.

When I come to that place of accepting my worst fears, when I stop resisting them and, instead, rest in them, I experience that it is not as bad as my mind had imagined. I used to think I would rather die than have persistent nausea. But when I rest in it and breathe with it, it's not so bad. I am showing up with the throwing up! It's not fun, but it's not horrendous either. It just is. I feel a stillness inside me as I surrender to it.

I am actually doing this cancer, chemo, radiation, nausea thing! I am doing it, and if I can do it, anyone can, though I hope you never have to. There is a beautiful song I once heard that repeats two words melodically over and over again throughout the song, "I surrender, I surrender, I surrender." I am singing that song.

When tear-streaked, little Emmy finally came out of

her torture chamber and walked by all of us compassionate witnesses in the waiting room, I wanted to reach out and hug her. Instead, I am hugging my own inner child who wants to resist reality, and I'm telling her, "I know this is scary. It's okay to feel scared. I'm sorry this is happening. I love you." She feels heard, she breathes, she starts to relax a bit. She shows up; and, to her surprise, she finds that it's not as bad as her fear had made it out to be.

Is there a part of you that is in pain, a part of you that is kicking and screaming and resisting reality? I invite you to move towards what you're feeling, meet yourself right where you are, and then give yourself a big hug. How brave we all are to be on this journey!

## 34

## COUNTING BLESSINGS
(June 5, 2010)

A good friend of mine recently returned home from a weekend trip with her husband and found that someone had broken into their house and stolen several pieces of expensive jewelry, including her wedding rings. At first she cried, but very quickly she shifted into acceptance and told me that I was the reason why. She said she thought about me and reasoned that she didn't have cancer, and no one died—that put things into perspective for her. She learned her lesson from the experience and was able to let it go.

That is a great illustration that how we choose to think about things affects our sense of wellbeing. It inspired me to focus on what I'm grateful for on this cancer journey, and I'd like to share some of it with you in this update.

About two weeks ago I had a CT scan which showed that my tumor is responding to the ongoing treatment. After four weeks, the 2" x 3" tumor shrunk to one fourth its original size. That is good news!

I am also grateful that for the last 2 weeks I haven't had chemo because my blood counts have been low. I needed a break from the relentless nausea and I got it. I'm using this reprieve to eat better, exercise more, and fortify my body.

This treatment could have been far worse. I haven't lost any hair! I haven't had to take narcotics as they'd said I might. Ibuprofen is handling the pain and discomfort.

I'm grateful that I'm in the homestretch—there are just three more days of radiation treatment and possibly one more chemo session, depending on my blood count. During these weeks of treatment, time has crawled like a snail. Now there is an end in sight. Yay!

Occasionally this fear comes up for me: what if this doesn't work? The doctor said that if the tumor doesn't completely disappear, it will grow back. When this fear appears, I've been doing the only thing I have control over—I've been training myself to come into the present. Throughout the day I say to myself, "Present moment, only moment." It is a blessing to be strengthening my ability to be fully present in the moment. It's a goal of mine in this lifetime, and feels like a huge accomplishment.

I am grateful for Tom who is taking such good care of me, and also himself and not letting himself become burned out. I am grateful for friends and family and the people who have been on this journey with me, giving me so much love and support.

I feel blessed that my cancer experience is being beneficial to some people, like my friend who put her loss into perspective and was able to let it go. People have told me that it has reminded them that life is precious and has inspired them to get more focused on what it is they're here to do, and what it is they really want. I feel honored and grateful to be of service in this way.

I am counting my many blessings. I am Here and Now. I am happy to be alive. There's always someone who has it worse off than us. My heart fills with compassion for them, and gratitude that I'm not them! It's all relative.

How about you? Counted your blessings lately? They really are plentiful when we look for them.

# 35

# I AM WILLING
(July 1, 2010)

My chemo and radiation treatments ended 3 weeks ago and tomorrow my doctor will examine me to see if the tumor is gone or still remains. The radiation continues to take effect 3 weeks after the treatment stops, so that's why the wait.

This waiting period has been a bit of a roller coaster ride. I've found myself fully in the Now at times, and at other times, I'm in the future where I sometimes imagine the worst and sometimes imagine the best. It's been difficult to think positive at times when I feel uncomfortable in my body, feeling my innards scorched by the radiation, feeling queasy and fatigued from chemo.

Right now I'm in a place of willingness. I am willing to be present with whatever comes up. I am willing to feel whatever feelings are here. I am willing to experience complete healing. I am willing to experience death. I am willing. What got me to this place was the realization that a part of me was NOT willing, a part of me was resisting and resenting.

Recently a friend of mine, who is very in touch with her light, has been exploring her shadows (those disowned parts of herself). She never thought she had shadows, so this is a new exploration for her. I started looking at how I see so clearly her shadows and her resistance to them, and I wondered if she was reflecting back to me something in myself that I've been resisting. As I told her, I believe that if it's in your life then it's in you. The people in our lives that push our buttons and stir our judgments are mirroring back to us our disowned parts. How nice of them! It helps me to remind myself that the goal is wholeness, and owning all my parts is what makes me whole.

I told my friend that a strong indicator that someone is reflecting back to us our disowned feelings is if we feel victimized by them (anger is often cleverly disguised as "victim"). As I explored this in myself, I was not aware of feeling victimized by anybody in my life, but I affirmed, "I am willing to see my shadows. I am willing to see every part of me. I am willing to be whole."

Just then it came to me...I don't feel victimized by anybody in my life...just my OWN body. I realized there is a part of me that feels let down by my body, disappointed, sad, mad, and scared. I did everything I could to be healthy, I ate well, took supplements, felt my feelings, connected with my spirit, loved myself and others, and yet I got cancer. I even ate mostly raw foods for a year and drank wheat grass juice every day after my hysterectomy; yet a lemon-sized tumor still grew in me in that year. Now I've been resisting taking supplements, thinking, what good did it do me? I'm seeing my cynicism, seeing that my surly Cynny persona has been operating from the shadows.

As I connect with the feeling of being betrayed by my body, I let myself cry and feel the disappointment and sadness. I ventilate my feelings, letting them move through me. I welcome my cynicism, disappointment. and sadness to the party. As I invite them out of the shadows into the light, I feel lighter, I feel more whole.

I've found that the best way to anchor myself in this place of wholeness, this place of openness and willingness to feel it all and be one with it all, is to 'TAG' myself. That's the acronym and practice I created over a year ago when I first discovered I had cancer. I wrote about it in an earlier essay, but I'll repeat it again here:

TAG – Trust, Acceptance, & Gratitude

I TRUST that I am loved, guided and watched over. I trust that things happen for a reason. I trust that my life is purposeful. I trust that everything will work out.

I ACCEPT that this is what's happening. It is what is. I breathe and allow it to be. This moment is perfect just as it is. I surrender to it. I become one with it.

I feel GRATITUDE for the many blessings in my life: my loving friends and family, my fellow journeyers and learning buddies, my wonderful husband Tom. I am grateful for this opportunity to cultivate more awareness, love, trust, and wholeness in my life. I am grateful that I remember that this is what is most important to me.

I feel scared to hear what my doctor has to say tomorrow; but I am willing to be present, to breathe, to feel my fear, and face whatever life presents to me. I am willing.

It is the next day and I just got back from my exam. The doctor said that there is still something there and it's about the same size that the last CT scan showed. The tumor shrunk to a quarter it's original size, but apparently did not shrink any more in the remaining weeks of treatment. He said that there's still a possibility that it could shrink more… or not. It could also grow back…or not. He suggested we wait and see and keep an eye on it. I don't foresee any further treatment.

So here I am, willing to be here one breath at a time. I think I'll go have a good cry, eat some chocolate, and then TAG myself again!

## 36

## JUICY NUGGETS
(July 11, 2010)

Last Wednesday I was interviewed about my cancer journey on Pamala Oslie's weekly radio show. Pamala is a high caliber psychic and author in Santa Barbara who receives my newsletters, felt inspired by them, and wanted me to share some of my learning with her listeners. I was nervous but also thrilled to think that sharing my experience and tools might help people. Being of service helps this whole thing make sense to me, it makes it all worth it.

Prior to the show, Pamala asked me to make a list of some of the things I'd be most excited talking about, my juiciest learning from this journey so far. Here's what I came up with:

TWO ARROWS
The Buddha talks about the two arrows of suffering. The first arrow is called primary suffering—it's when we have a physical pain or an emotional pain. The second arrow is called secondary suffering and it is self-inflicted when we react to the primary pain with resentment, resistance, distraction, or wallowing in victim energy. Those reactions lock the pain in. This has been a challenge of mine, to not get sucked into contractive victim energy. Finding ways to free myself of secondary suffering and move into expansive energy is one of my greatest challenges and most gratifying achievements. The following are valuable tools I'm using that might be helpful for you as well.

## A 'GOOD' CRY VS. A 'BAD' CRY

Since I found out last week that the chemo and radiation treatment didn't eliminate the cancer completely, I've felt scared and sad and have been having many a "good" cry. A good cry is when I feel the energy fully and allow it to pass through like a rain shower, and I feel clear and cleansed afterward. A "bad" cry is when I'm circling the drain in a sad story, round and round I go, and 'poor me' down the drain. A bad cry is very draining!

## BEFRIENDING THE FEELING

Sometimes I am gripped by fear. When that happens I move toward the fear by bringing my awareness to my body. I notice where I'm feeling the fear, such as shallow breath and a tight stomach. Then I name the feeling, saying, "I feel scared." No spin, no story, simply, "I feel scared." I begin to breath more easily. (This works with anger and sadness as well). Next I bring loving kindness to the fear, my Compassionate Witness talks to the fear, saying, "I know that you're scared. It's okay to feel scared. This is scary. I'm here with you. I love you. I'll take good care of you." More breath and more expansion happen. I'm now ready to TAG myself, affirming Trust, Acceptance, and Gratitude and I relax even more.

## IT IS WHAT IT IS

One of my greatest learnings in all this is to accept that this is what's happening. Accepting isn't giving up, it's coming into harmony with what is. It's letting go of the contractive energy of regret and resistance (secondary suffering), and coming into the expansive energy of surrender. That expansive energy leads to a state of grace where guidance and solutions appear. It's a state of flow where everything I need comes to me. It's a state of wholeness and oneness with all that is. It's a state of being where healing can happen.

## THE HEALING POWER OF PLAY

Singing, dancing, laughing and smiling creates endorphins, enhances the immune system and puts us in an expansive state. Reverend Michael Beckwith says that praying and playing are the same energetic. Chinese healer Chunyi Lin advocates that smiling generates healing love energy. He has a great acronym for SMILE: Starting My Internal Love Engine. Play is also a powerful shift tool when we're stuck in negative patterns. When I notice my cynical attitude is taking over, I play with it! I give it a name, Cynny, and I exaggerate her grousing, I let her rip! This brings her out of the shadows, into the light, into wholeness, and I expand into the playful, prayful state of grace. Plus, it's just plain fun!

## WAKE UP - YOUR DREAM IS WAITING TO BE BORN!

When I first found out I had uterine cancer just before my 60th birthday, having something growing in my uterus at the time of such an important birthday made me wonder, "What wants to be born into my life?" I realized that I had been stagnating—I'd done the same work for 27 years and was no longer inspired by it. I've always wanted to do inspirational writing. That was my dream. Cancer shook me awake and compelled me to take a risk and live my dream.

## GROWTH OPPORTUNITY

As someone on a spiritual path, I believe that life is all about soul growth and all about love. I see this cancer growth as the ultimate growth opportunity! I've asked myself, "What can I learn from this cancer? What wants to be loved here?" I see the tumor as an energy blockage and I ask myself, "How am I blocking my energy?" I realize that the belly and pelvic area of my body have sometimes been unloved parts of me. I haven't brought a lot of breath and awareness to the area. I've felt shame about some of the bodily functions there.

I've also blocked chi energy there by clenching in fear. I am now breathing fully into this area, ventilating it with healing energy. It has got my full loving attention.

THIS ETERNAL NOW MOMENT

Knowing that my time here may be limited has galvanized me into the present moment. I want to be fully here and now, fully alive while I am alive. I'm seeing the world through present-moment baby eyes, I am brand new and drinking it all in. Tom and I look into each other's eyes, really seeing each other, feeling the eternity of the present moment. When I find myself thinking about the future and worrying, I affirm, "Present moment, only moment." When I'm fully in the present, time actually expands and it's beautiful. In truth, right now is all there is. I am here now. "It is eternity now; I am in the midst of it. It is about me in the sunshine; I am in it, as the butterfly in the light-laden air. Nothing has to come; it is now. Now is eternity; now is immortal life."-(Richard Jefferies)

It is such an honor and so gratifying to me that my writing about this cancer experience may be of help to people in some way. I truly feel that I am right where I'm supposed to be. I am doing my soul's work. I relax in the knowing that this moment is perfect just as it is.

How about you? If you could sum up the juicy nuggets gathered from the challenges in your life, what would they be?

# 37

## A STATE OF GRACE PLACE
(August 3, 2010)

I've been hanging out in a state of grace place. It's the expanded energy field, the natural order of harmony and wholeness. It's a place you go to when you pray, when you connect with your higher power and ask for divine intervention.

It is a transcendent place beyond mind, beyond reason, beyond physical, beyond what most doctors will tell you is possible. My oncologist told me last week that though my tumor has been reduced in size, it will start growing again because that's what tumors do—end of story. But in the state of grace place it's not the end of the story. Miracles happen there. Healing happens there.

I'm reminded of Dr. Leonard Laskow's fascinating experiments with cancer cells in petri dishes in which he held an intention as he focused on each dish. The intention that had the most success in stopping the growth of the cancer cells by 39% was when he affirmed and imagined, "The natural order is being reinstated and the cells growth is returning to normal." I am motivated to focus on and cultivate that state of natural order and harmony, not only because I want to heal, but also because it feels good—it is a peaceful, magical place.

Being in a state of grace is being in the flow where synchronicity occurs, coincidences happen, just the right people, books, and events present themselves, and things work out better than I can imagine. It is the realm of unlimited possibilities. I also refer to it as the Miracle-Prone Zone.

I was recently stuck in the Moan and Groan Zone, feeling ravaged by the grueling chemo and radiation treatment. I realized that Cynny, my inner cynical one, was feeling burned out and pissy and she was keeping me down. She was cynical about taking healthful actions—after all, she groused, they didn't work before. Yet I knew that underneath the cynicism was a fear that if I tried and failed to heal myself I would be crushed in disappointment. I realized that I needed help.

As I cultivated the state of grace place, I was 'led' to a coach who has guided people for 20 years on conscious cancer journeys. (Her name is Melanie Brown, her website is consciouscancerjourney.com) My commitment to working with her helped get me back to a healing intention of eating healthy foods, taking supplements and, most important, shifting my attitude and letting myself believe that I could heal myself.

Next, in the flow of synchronicity, a friend sent me a link about antiangiogenesis foods that actually starve tumors, either causing them to shrink or halting further growth by eliminating their blood supply. I am now eating those foods abundantly with a new sense of hope and possibility. (See list in Chapter 48 - Healing Regimen and Resources)

This exciting grace place where anything is possible is where I want to live. However, though this place is becoming home base, I'm not always here. I take occasional forays to the rat race place where I'm scared, scrambling, and frantic. The other day hundreds of ants had gathered in and around our cat's food dish and I set about attacking the ants with the fervor of a mass murderer! It reminded me of the fear frenzy I sometimes feel towards the cancer.

However, when I notice I'm not breathing and my shoulders are hunched and my stomach is tight and I'm feeling like it's me against THEM, I take a deep breath and return to my home base state of grace, where natural order and peace are reinstated.

Taking deep, slow breaths is one of the ways to enter a state of grace. Other ways are meditation, reading inspirational books, doing qigong, dancing, being with spiritual people, dropping into stillness and silence, being immersed in the present moment, walking in nature (a natural tuning fork for raising your vibration), laughing and playing, and cuddling with my husband Tom as we breathe together and reveal ourselves in deep intimacy.

I am a gardener gardening my energy field, raising my consciousness, choosing to dwell in a state of grace. It's the place to be. It feels like Home. From all that I've heard about death, it is the ultimate state of grace place. If I'm going Home soon, I'm getting a good taste of it (and for it) right now as I nestle into the welcoming embrace of grace. It's possible that I may not be cured, but I will be healed and made whole. Of that I am certain.

What are ways you enter your state of grace place? I am wishing for all of you (and me) the magic and miracles that take place when we rest in the loving embrace of grace.

# 38

## FREEDOM!
### (August 15, 2010)

I recently watched a new TV show called "The Big C" about a reserved woman, played by wonderful actress Laura Linney, who suddenly learns she has terminal cancer. She realizes that time is precious and this sets her free to change her life, to assert herself and do things she'd been too afraid and uptight to do. In a restaurant she declares, "I'm just having desserts and liquor."

I've been experiencing a similar freedom. The thought that death could possibly be just around the corner liberates me to live with a certain amount of abandon. As the song says, "Freedom's just another word for nothing left to lose." I am free to not sweat the small stuff, to do only what I want to do, to focus on raising my vibration and living in the state of grace that I love so much.

Even though a part of me wants to really let loose and eat gooey desserts and drink liquor like Laura Linney's character, I know that would debilitate my health (cancer loves sugar!) and knock me out of the state of grace place. I'm motivated by my belief that I can heal myself, or at least prolong my life; so instead of eating desserts and drinking liquor, I am eating lots of anti-cancer foods and drinking an herbal tea from my Chinese Medicine doctor that looks and tastes like it was scraped off the forest floor! I hold my nose when I drink it, and as I drink I affirm to myself, "This is powerful, healing medicine."

James Dean said, "Dream as if you'll live forever. Live

as if you'll die tomorrow." I am dreaming and eating as if I'll live forever and I am living and loving as if I'll die tomorrow. I feast my eyes and soul on the beauty that surrounds me, the summer flowers, the Santa Barbara mountains, and the beautiful people in my life. I don't think I'd be enjoying such a feast if it weren't for the cancer…or, as I am choosing to call it, "The burr under my saddle that woke me up."

As friends from out of town stop by and visit with me, I know that it's possible it may be the last time I see them. (That is true for all of us. Who knows what life will bring?) Therefore, I really see and appreciate them and savor being in their presence and when we say goodbye to each other, there is a depth and a sweetness to it.

I am valuing each moment. Whenever I think about death, I'm reminded that I am alive now. I am here now. Here and now is all there is. In this here and now I'm choosing to raise my vibration and let my light shine. At the end of the first episode of The Big C, the song that plays is, "This little light of mine, I'm gonna let it shine. Let it shine, let it shine, let it shine." That sums it all up perfectly. We are free at any time to fully allow our light to shine.

If you thought you might only have a short time to live, how would you let your light shine? What dream of yours would you be living? Do it now—"Dream as if you'll live forever. Live as if you'll die tomorrow."

## 39

# THE UNIVERSE IS GOOSING ME!
## (August 29, 2010)

"Our cells are constantly eavesdropping on our thoughts and being changed by them." I love that quote by Deepak Chopra. It reminds me to be aware of my thoughts and the reality they are creating. Science has shown that our cells can literally rearrange themselves according to our thoughts and attitudes. Our cells await our direction, and in the meantime they operate on old habitual programming.

The cancer coach I'm working with, Melanie Brown, is providing me with tools that help me to intentionally create the life and state of being that I want. One of the tools is called Scripting, which involves taking time each morning to write down how I desire my day to go, to see my day and my health in positive possibilities as if it were already so. The physical act of writing these desires builds new neural pathways, and my cells 'eavesdrop' on these affirmations and arrange themselves accordingly.

When I've done the scripting, my day has unfolded remarkably close to the script I laid out for that day. However, I was new to scripting and hadn't made it a habit yet, and I started to forget to do it. Without conscious direction, old thought habits were starting to creep in.

I recently awoke constricted in fear with a pain in my butt that had been aching throughout the night. This dull aching pain had been persistent lately. It is the same pain I'd once mistook for hemorrhoids, but my doctor told me that it is most probably referred pain from the site of the tumor.

I'd been hoping that all my healing efforts were succeeding in eliminating or holding the cancer at bay (and that may be true, the pain could simply be referred pain from scar tissue from the radiation). However, fear of the worst-case scenario had me in its grip.

I fell into Tom's arms as the 'rains' came, crying, and expressing my feelings and my worst fears. One of those is that I will die a painful, lingering death. I'm not afraid of death itself, but, as Woody Allen said, "I just don't want to be there when it happens." As I cried and acknowledged this fear, a clearing happened—the fear loosened its grip and the pain lessened, giving me the direct experience that fear makes the pain worse. When I'm tense and barely breathing, the pain increases which makes me more tense, which makes the pain intensify, and so on until before I know it I'm all crunched up in a black hole of fear and pain.

I was feeling better and pain-free from ventilating my feelings, and continued to process with Tom. I told him that I've been thinking about going to a medical intuitive because I realize a part of me wants someone to see my energy field and recognize and acknowledge the value of my soul's journey. I said to Tom, "I wonder what words I would love to hear her say? What higher truth would I love for her to see about me and this health challenge?" I imagined I was the medical intuitive telling me everything I'd love to hear. Here's what 'she' told me:

"I see that you are a strong, courageous soul, facing your worst fears, making a stand in this lifetime to heal and integrate all of your unloved parts. I see your passion to become whole. I also see that you've already done a lot of work on yourself, healing yourself in many ways, and, now there is this one area that needs your loving attention. You are right where you're supposed to be. You are loving yourself whole, and you are doing a great job!"

It's natural for us to want all our hard work to be

seen, and to have our magnificent Soul Self recognized and acknowledged by others…and, I realize that it's most important that I recognize and acknowledge that about myself. Therefore, I've decided to include in my daily scripting an appreciation for the magnificence of my Big Soul Self.

During the day, if there is pain, I now use it to alert me that I've contracted into the little, fearful, pain-in-the-butt me, and that reminds me to breathe, relax and return to the awareness of my Magnificent Big Ass Soul Self! The pain is like the Universe goosing me, saying, "Unclench, breathe, stay awake and remember who you really are. Remember that you are loved and watched over. Remember that you are eternal. Remember that you are safe no matter what." When I'm in that place of remembrance, I breathe easy, I relax, and the pain lessens or completely disappears.

One of my favorite passages from Bartholomew's book, *I Come As a Brother*, is about putting fear into perspective. He says, "It is as though you injured your little finger but the rest of your body is all right…Isolate the fear into your 'finger' and call on the whole 'body' to clarify it." I'm seeing the cancer in the same way—I'm putting it into perspective. It is not who I am, it is not all of me, it is not bigger than me; it's just a little bitty baby burr under my saddle reminding me to WAKE UP!

At this time I don't know if the remaining tumor is shrinking, growing, spreading or staying the same. I know that I feel good physically (except for the occasional pain in the butt, which has lessened considerably). I am recovering from the chemo and radiation and I'm feeling more strength and vitality every day. I have been scripting for that and it is so. I've now made the scripting a habitual part of my day and it has made a big difference in my sense of wellbeing, happiness and health.

Fear has been a 'pain in the butt' for me in this lifetime. I am facing and embracing it and using it to remind me that we are so much more than our bodies—we are big, bright, beautiful, eternal souls here to learn and grow and remember that we are big, bright, beautiful, eternal souls.

What script would you write for your ideal day? If someone could see who you really are—all your brilliance, all your hard work—what words of acknowledgement would you love to hear them say? Say them to yourself! Script them into your day. Then 'goose' yourself to stay awake and keep remembering all day long how magnificent, courageous and valuable you truly are!

## 40

## LIFE IS A WONDERFUL ADVENTURE
(September 5, 2010)

Each morning when we let our kitties out, I watch them step cautiously over the threshold of the door, with their heads lowered, crouching as they look around the porch for hidden dangers. "Where is dat big black meany cat? Do yu see dat orange cat dat messes wid us?" They are scared but they want to go outside anyway and experience the great adventure that is life.

I am thrilled that we sprung the kitties from their safe prison (they were indoor cats for their first four years) and released them to the pleasures and terrors of the outside world. It's so much fun watching them taste all of life, including rats, and having exciting explorations and glorious adventures.

"Life is where one goes to temporarily believe in death, fleetingly forget their power, and briefly have the Dickens scared out of them, voluntarily. All in the name of adventure."-(Mike Dooley) Life is a wonderful adventure and it is sometimes very scary, but oh so worth it—especially when we remember our power.

This morning I was reminded of that power. Tom held me in his arms and told me how much he loved having me in his life, how he loved my body and my soul, loved all of who I am and felt lucky to be with me. I took it in, marveling at this miracle in my life—a miracle I intentionally created.

For many years I longed to hear those words from someone, but I didn't really believe I ever would. I remember when Santa Barbara psychic Pamala Oslie told me about Tom years before he appeared in my life, describing him perfectly and saying, "He thinks you're wonderful. He thinks you're beautiful." That was very hard for me to believe, and that was the problem—I needed to believe those things about myself before he could come into my life. I also needed to be willing to step over the threshold into the scary, exciting adventure that is love.

One day I decided that I was ready to take on that great adventure. I proclaimed to myself, "I am willing to do whatever it takes." I was finally willing to face all the fears that relationship brought up for me, the terror of possible pain and abandonment, the fear of loss. I was willing to heal my heart and open to love.

I turned all my energy and focus towards that mission, that great adventure of loving and being loved. I saturated my life with that purpose, I marinated in that goal, I passionately focused on it, and the Universe responded by bringing me everything I needed for that great journey, including Tom!

Now, in present time, lying in Tom's arms, I thought to myself, "Wouldn't it be great to create another miracle, a healing miracle? I healed the blockage in my heart...I can heal this blockage in my pelvic area in the same way."

I have stepped over the threshold into this cancer adventure and it is scary, exciting and awakening. I am willing to do whatever it takes to get the fullest learning and healing from this experience. I am marinating myself in love, healing energy, vibrant foods, and high vibrations. Consequently the universe is flowing to me everything I need in order to heal: inspiring books, topnotch healers, and love and prayers from the beautiful people in my life. In the midst of cancer, I often feel a sense of ease, trust and wellbeing—I call that a miracle!

How about you? Is there a threshold beckoning you to step over it? Do you remember the power you possess to create the scary, exciting, enlivening life of your dreams? I am wishing for you a wonderful adventure!

# 41

## FORGIVENESS
(September 29, 2010)

As part of my focus on deep healing, I'm reading a book called *The Cancer Cleanse*, which advocates that one of the most important things that needs to be cleansed is our energy around forgiveness, or rather unforgiveness. Holding onto emotional hurts creates an acidic state in the body, making it a breeding ground for cancer growth and other illnesses. It's made me wonder if there are people I need to forgive.

I'm reading another book called *Journey of Souls* by Michael Newton. He is a hypnotherapist who has regressed thousands of people to the life-between-life state. Most people report that after they die they are welcomed by loved ones on the other side, often by their deceased parents. They exclaim, "Oh, there's my beloved mother and father. How wonderful to see them again!" I sadly realized that I wouldn't have that reaction to seeing my mother and father. I have a frozen image of my mother as a cold, refrigerator mom, and my father as a volatile, volcano dad.

Even though I'd thought that through all my years of personal growth work I'd forgiven them and accepted them as they were, I can see that my mind has locked them into those limited images. I know they were more than a fridge and a volcano, but unforgiveness is insidiously one-dimensional. It locks in the bad image of people and locks out anything good about them.

When I was diagnosed with cancer and was about to send out my first newsletter about it, I was estranged from one of my longtime best friends. We'd had a fight and hadn't spoken to each other for a couple months. In my mind she was the devil—I couldn't remember what I'd ever liked about her. She was seeing me in that same negative light. It is so scary to me how our minds can obliterate, eviscerate, and eliminate others like that, especially someone who has been so close to us.

But cancer softened me, it got me out of my steel-trap mind and into my broken-open heart and loosened the grip of unforgiveness. I decided to include her on my newsletter list (she was not aware that I had been diagnosed with cancer). As I pressed the button to send it out, in that same second I received an email from her! She wrote that she had a foreboding sense that something bad might have happened to me and wanted me to know that despite our differences she still loved me and wanted to know if I was all right.

That blew my mind and melted my heart. It was amazing to me that we had reached out to each other SIMULTANEOUSLY! It shows how connected we are to the important people in our lives. As we reentered each other's lives, I remembered how much I loved her. She has brought a richness and joy to my life that I would not be experiencing if I hadn't moved beyond my frozen image of her. What a terrible loss that would have been.

A life-threatening illness is one way to shift us out of our closed mind into our open heart, but there are less drastic ways. My husband Tom told me that one of his mentors, Dick Olney, sometimes worked with people on their memories of their parents. He had them vividly imagine their parents the way they would've liked them to be, to really get into seeing and feeling it as if it were actually so. This helped melt the frozen image their minds were fixated on and allowed memories to flow of things they liked about their parents. The story they'd been stuck in was changed forever and they were free to have a new experience of their parents.

My cancer coach told me about another 'unfreezing'

technique: think of the person we are having a hard time forgiving and ask ourselves, "How would God (or our Higher Self) see this person?" Forgiveness isn't a one-time thing—it's a continual work in progress. I realize there are things I'm still forgiving myself for, like my own moments of fire and ice, times of volcanic eruptions and glacial reserve. What helps me most is to see myself from the sweet perspective and unconditional love of my Higher Self, to feel compassion for myself and know that I'm doing the best that I can.

I see that this is true about my parents as well, and this expands my limited view of them. I'm remembering that there was lots of playfulness, laughter and good times. I'm remembering that they did the best that they could. I'm remembering that they are a part of me and I am a part of them. Michael Newton says that in his work regressing people to their life-between-life states he's found that we actually CHOOSE our parents for all the learning and growth that they spur in us.

Ultimately, I know that the most important healing for me in this lifetime is not healing cancer…it is healing the feeling of being wronged, and melting my frozen negative images of others. I'm seeing it all as part of the plan to grow myself to wholeness, and learning to see myself and others the way God would.

I've learned that when I build a case against others, I become imprisoned in that case. I am the one who is freed when I forgive—it is so much more fun and spacious living in an open heart than a closed mind. That's where I'm aiming to be.

Are there people in your life you want to forgive? Ask yourself, "How does God see this person?" And when you need to forgive yourself, ask, "How does God see me?" Then serenade yourself with Joe Cocker's song, "You Are So Beautiful to Me."

## 42

# THE HEALING POWER OF IKIGAI
(October 10, 2010)

My conscious cancer coach has asked me some very profound questions, such as: what is keeping you here, what is your passion, what engages you and gives your life purpose? In other words, what is my ikigai?

Ikigai (sounds like icky guy) is a Japanese word that basically means 'why I wake up in the morning'. It's what brings meaning and joy to our lives. The reason those questions are so important is because the answers could make a difference between healing or not healing, life or death. Studies have found that people who have discovered their ikigai live longer, happier, healthier lives. Our ikigai could be our children, work, plants or pets—anything that we care for and care about. Its healing power comes from taking our focus off our problems and instead focusing us on what we love. This turns off destructive stress hormones and activates healing energy.

A good friend recently sent me this sweet letter:

"My cat Merlin, my little furry man, had a cancer tumor taken off last year...the vet didn't seem optimistic. He lost lots of weight and I was giving up on him. He still had an appetite so I fed him as often as he wanted, tuna, salmon, shrimp, but he still didn't gain a pound. In the last few months instead of fretting, I just started to enjoy him, take his fleas off twice a day and tell him how beautiful and wonderful he is. He gets on the sink 3 or 4 times a day waiting to be told how wonderful he is and I groom him a little. Its 8 months later and his coat and weight are getting back to normal." My friend stopped worrying and just focused on loving and nurturing his cat and it was healing for both of them.

Here are some additional examples of the miraculous healing effects of focusing on what we love:

When Phoebe Snetsinger was diagnosed with terminal cancer, she decided to follow her bliss and travel the world sighting birds. Her cancer went into remission and she lived twenty more years, and set the world's record for sighting the most bird species ever.

Ten years ago my brother Norm was diagnosed with an inoperable brain aneurysm. He eventually stopped thinking about the time bomb in his head and focused on fulfilling his dream of sailing his boat to the Caribbean Islands and beyond. He was recently told by doctors that an MRI showed the aneurysm had calcified and was no longer a problem.

My acupuncturist told me about a woman he was treating with stage 4 cancer whose doctors could do no more for her and told her to check into hospice. When he asked her if there was something she loved to do, she remembered her love of painting that she'd given up years ago due to a busy life. She took up painting again and her cancer disappeared.

They all focused on what they loved doing and their illness subsided. Our ikigai can heal what ails us, AND what ails us can awaken us to our ikigai.

I believe there are possible exit points OR step up points in our lives; times when we decide to renew or not renew our contract with life; times we ask ourselves, "Am I having fun? Do I still want to be here? Is there something I'd love to do and am I willing to do it?"

When I was a depressed, suicidal teenager I was faced with these questions. My depression led me to reading metaphysical books like *The Power of Positive Thinking*, *Your Thoughts Can Change Your Life* and *Psycho-Cybernetics*. I became very excited and deeply resonated with what these books were saying. I knew my thoughts and feelings created my reality and I wanted to take on the challenge of transforming my life. This gave me a reason to live—it became my ikigai and fueled amazing transformation and healing over the years.

When I was approaching my 50th birthday, I was feeling bored with life and uninspired. I became aware that it was a possible exit point...or a step up point. Someone I knew had just died of an illness at age 50. It seemed that she had given up and was choosing to check out. I realized that my stagnation could possibly lead to something like that happening.

I checked in with myself and realized I wasn't ready to leave this life. I wanted to stick around and face one of my biggest life challenges—creating a conscious, loving relationship. That was my new ikigai. I passionately immersed myself in that pursuit, AND, an anything but icky guy showed up...the wondrous Tom!

Now, some ten years later, I am faced with another possible exit point or step up point—within the past two years my appendix ruptured and then cancer came a callin'. I am seriously addressing the questions my cancer coach posed to me: Do I still want to be here? Is there something I feel passionate about doing? Are there exciting challenges that are engaging me?

The answer is yes. My relationship with my husband Tom continues to be a great joy and something I dearly love. Cancer has refocused me on additional passions and reasons for living, like writing, and deeply connecting with my spirit. It has renewed my enthusiasm for metaphysics, exploring how our thoughts and feelings affect our reality, our bodies, and our lives. As I'm working on healing myself, I'm highly engaged in reading stimulating books such as *Spontaneous Healing of Belief* by Gregg Braden, and *The*

*Intention Experiment* by Lynne McTaggert. Science has now caught up with metaphysics and it's a very exciting time to be alive.

Gardening is an ikigai for many people and in a sense it is for me as well. I am now passionately focused on gardening my energy field, gardening a higher vibration, gardening the healing energy of love. Like my friend who stopped worrying and simply showered love on his cat, I am loving myself, I am lovingly talking to my body and my ailing parts like they're my children, telling them how wonderful and beautiful they are. I am loving delicious food and delicious connections with the people in my life. I look forward to waking up in the morning, fully tasting and enjoying life. These are all exciting, worthwhile reasons to be here.

"When you wake up in the morning, Pooh," said Piglet, "what's the first thing you say to yourself?" "What's for breakfast?" said Pooh. "What do you say, Piglet?" "I say, I wonder what's going to happen exciting today?" said Piglet. Pooh nodded thoughtfully. "It's the same thing," he said.

I believe our ikigai is a key element in whether we stay or go, whether we kick the bucket or keep filling the bucket. I want to stay. I want to keep filling the bucket!

What's your ikigai? What are you excited about and motivates you to jump out of bed in the morning? It could be something as simple as breakfast (like Pooh) or something as profound as loving and nurturing yourself as if you were the most precious thing in the world. I wish you buckets full of ikigai!

## 43

## ONE WITH EVERYTHING
(October 25, 2010)

Right now I don't know what the state of my cancer is, and I don't want to know. Not knowing helps keep me focused on hope and healing. For the most part I feel fine, I am going about my life, doing my alternative treatments, and thinking that maybe I'm going to be okay. I've taken up residence in the miracle-prone zone, visualizing health and wholeness. There's a bumper sticker that says, "Expect miracles." I am expecting a miracle—that is, most of me is…then there's the rest of me.

That's the thing about not knowing for sure. There are times when I think I might be whistling in the dark, fooling myself, and I wonder if I'm living in a miracle or a mirage? Sometimes I'll be going along doing just fine, then something happens that triggers a flood of fear and sadness as the awareness hits me, "I have cancer."

I recently went to Pizza Guru (One with Everything) and had an unexpected melt down. I was happy to find a pizza place that used whole-wheat crust. I've been staying away from white foods like bread, rice and pasta because when eaten they quickly turn into sugar, which feeds cancer. But when I arrived to pick up my pizza, I realized I'd forgotten to specify whole-wheat crust and my pizza had white crust. I told the girl, "I can't eat white," and suddenly tears started rolling down my face. The poor girl thought I was crying about white crust, when actually I was struck with the deep sadness that I may have a terminal illness.

As they were making me a new pizza with whole-wheat crust, I sat in the sanctuary of my car and let the dam burst—I sobbed and sobbed and sobbed. It felt so good to let it out. Feeling purged, clarity, peace and calm followed and I became One with everything. Like Seth says, "Any feeling fully felt and experienced always leads you back to love."

I recently joined a women's empowerment group, which is a way to state my intention to the universe that I want to be here, on this planet, in this earth suit known as Janet, to continue learning, growing, healing and helping. At the first meeting, I held back sharing my circumstances with them, afraid that once I named it I'd be swept away in a river of tears. When I told them, sure enough the floods came, but passed through quickly, and once again I came to a place of calm strength.

Some people say you need to be 100% positive in order to manifest the positive results you want. They say don't even think about cancer, don't envision it, don't give it energy. I can understand that reasoning, I know that what we focus on grows. But, at the same time, what we resist persists, and completely ignoring it turns it into the boogey man. Trying to wall it off and will it away is like pushing down a Jack-in-the-Box that will eventually POP UP with a big bad BOO! Or a big sad BOO HOO!

There are others, like Abraham Hicks and Bartholomew, who say that all you need is to be 51% positive, and that shifts the balance into an optimistic view and outcome. I can do that—I can do 51%. I'm learning that I can also welcome whatever feelings want to pop up, stop in, and pass through, even the big boo's and boo-hoos. I trust that the fears and tears I thought might drown me DO move through easily when I allow them free passage, without resistance and story, bringing me to an empowered place of wholeness.

With Halloween approaching, it's the perfect time for embracing our shadows, to bring them into the light and play with them. It's a great time to dress up as our worst fears and our disowned parts, including our brilliance. Maybe I'll dress up as a ravenous tumor, or the Grim Reaper, or the Queen of Denial, or...as a Pizza, ONE with Everything.

Do you have feelings that you fear will engulf you if you let them out? I encourage you to invite them to the party, welcome your worst fears and highest aspirations and announce yourself as, "Party of ONE!"

## 44

## TRANSFORMING WITH YES SETS
(November 22, 2010)

Right now I feel really good. I am pain-free for the first time in a year. I am feeling happy, peaceful and healthy. No, this isn't me reciting pie-in-the-sky affirmations about how I want it to be…it is actually SO! Despite the doctors prediction that my cancer will inevitably grow and that basically I'm toast, I'm still here and I'm feeling better all the time. Could it be that something I'm doing is working?!

I'm not sure exactly what that might be since I'm doing a multitude of healing modalities. However, I am convinced that one of the most powerful things I am doing is called 'Yes Sets'. Yes Sets have a proven track record in my life of producing miracles.

What are Yes Sets? They are a form of hypnosis which involves saying a series of persuasive truisms that get your head nodding and mind agreeing and affirming, "Yes, that's true." This activates the agreement part of our brain. Then at the end of this series of at least three true statements, you slip in the desired, related belief. Yes Sets help set us up for new, desired possibilities, and set us free from stubborn, habitual mindsets. The reason this is important is that the mind has tremendous influence over what plays out in our bodies and in our lives. Our life and our body are shaped and formed by our thoughts and beliefs.

A perfect example of this is the amazing, true account of "Mr. Wright" (a pseudonym), who in the mid 1950's was dying from cancer of the lymph nodes. He had tumors the size of oranges and was weak and feverish and clearly on his way out. His doctors gave him an experimental drug called Krebiozen. Within a few days his tumors were half their size and ten days later they were almost completely gone and he was restored to good health.

However, when he heard reports that the drug was a failure, his health declined and his tumors returned. His doctors decided to try an experiment. They told him those reports were wrong, that the drug actually did work at a higher dosage. This time they gave him a placebo, telling him it was a higher dose of Krebiozen, and once again his tumors vanished and he returned to good health. Alas, a few months later the AMA came out with a formal announcement that the drug was useless, and shortly thereafter Mr. Wright checked into a hospital and died of his disease.

The mind can kill us or cure us. Convincing the mind that what we want IS possible is paramount and Yes Sets are a powerful way to accomplish that. I'll give you an example of the miraculous mind and life altering effect of using Yes Sets in my life. Most of my life I had a deeply entrenched belief that I was unlovable and would always be alone. I literally could not conceive of being loved by a man. When I finally figured out that that was simply a hard-wired habitual belief, I began using Yes Sets to change that belief. Here is one of the Yes Sets I used that evoked an affirmative response and helped open my mind, and therefore my life, to love:

*There's plenty of blue sky for everyone.*
*There's plenty of oxygen for everyone.*
*There's plenty of love for everyone.*
*There's plenty of love for me.* (This desired belief easily slips into the series of yeses preceding it).

Another set of persuasive truisms that I used were:

*I am a valuable friend with depth, humor and a commitment
to authenticity and personal growth.*
*My friends deeply love and appreciate that about me.*
*I deeply love and appreciate that about myself.*
*There are men who would love to have a partner with those
qualities.*
*There are men who would love to have me as a partner.*
*In fact, some man would be dang lucky to have me as a
partner!*

By using Yes Sets (and other techniques), I successfully
convinced myself that I was lovable, that I deserved love
and could have a lasting, loving relationship with the man of
my dreams. Soon love came into my life in the form of my
husband-to-be, Tom, who is a constant visual reminder to me
that hardwired beliefs can be changed, and deeply desired
beliefs can become reality.

Now, as I'm healing from cancer, I'm affirming a series
of affirmative, head-nodding truisms such as:

*I am daily, diligently doing powerful healing modalities.*
*These modalities have produced miraculous cures for many
people.*
*Miracles happen in my life.*
*I am feeling stronger and healthier everyday.*
*I believe these modalities can produce a miraculous cure for
me.*
*I believe that I can be completely healed!*

As I dwell in these truisms I have come to believe that
maybe I will be around for a while. Maybe I'm not toast
after all. Maybe I'll be the toast of the town! Maybe I really
will be completely healed! I know that this belief rearranges

my cells, my reality and my outcome. As Deepak Chopra has written, "We are the only creatures on the planet who can change our biology through our thoughts, feelings and intentions. Our cells are constantly eavesdropping on our thoughts and being changed by them."

Do you have a hardwired belief that you would like to change? Is there something you would like to have in your life but believe it's impossible? I highly recommend using Yes Sets to help set you free from old programming and set you up for unlimited possibilities. Yes! Yes! Yes!

## 45

# CHRISTMAS 'MIRROR-CLE'
(December 20, 2010)

"Mirrors, mirrors all around, reflections of myself abound. What most needs to be loved is found in what I judge in you."

That's from a poem I wrote about projection a few years ago. Along the same lines, there's a saying that goes, "If you spot it, you got it." It means that what we see and judge in others is in us in some way.

Having cancer and not knowing how much longer I have (do any of us really?), I am compelled to clean up my act as much as possible; to face my shadows, free myself of judgments, heal, and become whole. I'm feeling healthy, but recently discovered a hard, pea-sized bump under my skin that could be a giant pimple OR a life-threatening tumor (which would mean the cancer is spreading). I don't know if I'm making a mountain out of a molehill, a tumor out of a pimple, but either way, it is a burr under my saddle (yes, it is located in THAT region once again) spurring me to own my projections and make peace with those aspects of myself being reflected back to me in other people.

This is an ongoing work in progress. Though I'd love to be completely free of judgments…alas, saint I ain't (as Tom's father used to say). Just when I think I got all my wacky, quacky ducks in a row and feel like I'm doing pretty darn good spiritually, the universe sends me people who push my buttons and I am once again confronted with my judgments.

Some of you might be currently experiencing this if you're visiting family during this holiday season because, as Ram Dass once said, "If you think you are enlightened, go visit your family."

I had a profound learning about projections a number of years ago while visiting my family at my childhood home—what I like to call the 'button factory' because that's where all my buttons were installed. I considered these visits my yearly exam where I could put to the test all my latest self-help tools. Things would go really well...for the first hour or two, sometimes even a day or two; but then, sure enough, my mom would criticize or hover and my buttons would be activated, and I'd be lost in the button factory.

One time during one of these visits, after a difficult day, I awoke in the middle of the night with an epiphany...I imagined my family asleep in their rooms and in the quiet space of the night I saw my mother's critical nature, and I realized that I have a critical nature. I thought about my brother and how easily offended he could be and thought, "Oh, I'm easily offended." I took a good look at my sister's people pleaser and realized that I'm a people pleaser at times.

Everything I judged in them was in me. I had been judging in them what I hadn't wanted to face in myself. It wasn't just an intellectual awareness of it; it was a full body, full spirit experience of our interconnectedness. Instead of seeing me versus them, I was seeing me as them, and them as me. I experienced that we were part of the same whole and were reflections of each other. I had to smile to myself when I really got that they were my mirrors—it was a 'mirror-cle' moment!

I realize that the real test in life isn't seeing how long I can go without my buttons being pushed—the real test is being able to face and embrace all of the disowned, projected parts of me. It's not about becoming perfect—it's about becoming whole by loving and accepting all the many me's that life is reflecting back to me: the meany me's, the moody me's, the messy me's, and even the mighty me's.

Sometimes in the early morning I'll look at my sleeping husband Tom and I'll think to myself, "Wow, if everyone in my life is my mirror, then Tom is my mirror and I think Tom is wonderful, I think Tom is a beautiful soul." I have many beautiful souls in my life (including my family) and since they are my mirrors, I must be a beautiful soul too. Being able to face and embrace THAT is truly the biggest mirror-cle of all!

Are there people in your life who are pushing your buttons? What are they mirroring in you that you haven't owned? Do you have beautiful souls in your life? That's because you are one! Mirrors, mirrors all around, reflections of yourself abound! I'm wishing for you the Christmas mirror-cle of loving all the many hues of the many you's reflected in your life.

REFLECTIONS OF ONE

*What I think are enemies*
*are really just the many me's,*
*projected out identities*
*for me to see and love.*

*Some will shout obscenities,*
*some without amenities.*
*All seem to be them, not me,*
*yet all are mine to love.*

*Mirrors mirrors all around,*
*reflections of myself abound.*
*What most needs to be loved is found*
*in what I judge in you.*

*Loving is the alchemy*
*that transforms you and me to we,*
*the 'mirror-cle' that helps me see*
*that we are really ONE.*
-Janet Jacobsen

## 46

# THE BLESSING OF BORROWED TIME
(January 15, 2011)

Good news—what I thought was a possible tumor (and spreading cancer) turned out to be just a large pimple after all! However, it served as a reminder that I am living on borrowed time, and also reminded me that my situation is not grave…it's gravy! Faced with possible imminent death, I am fully appreciating and tasting each moment and experiencing that time has magically slowed and expanded. As I'm immersed in the present, savoring it, I'm finding that this present is the gift that keeps on giving.

After the chemo and radiation treatment failed to completely eliminate my tumor nearly 8 months ago, I thought I was a goner, I thought my days were numbered… and not a big number at that. I had a dental cleaning around that time and didn't know if I'd be around for the next cleaning in 6 months. I wasn't sure if I should even make an appointment. But next month it's time for the cleaning and I am still here, feeling healthy and enjoying this groovy gravy grateful time!

My husband Tom told me that his father lived with that grateful attitude each and every day, ever since an incident that happened when he was a young man serving in World War II. One day during the war, he generously gave up his foxhole to another man and sought shelter elsewhere. The man in the foxhole was killed by an artillery shell. After that Tom's father believed that there was nothing to worry about because from then on life was a gift, it was all gravy.

I'm feeling that too. Even though it is so strange not knowing what is happening in my body with the cancer—is it stable, or on the move, or completely gone?!—I feel alert, awake, happy to be alive, wanting to learn all that I can while I'm still here on schoolhouse Earth, and feeling inspired to share what I'm learning.

I also feel a great lessening of the fear that had gripped me before. I have accepted death and the possible pain involved, and have come to a place of peace with it all, a 'bring it!" place. I know that I can do this. I can face whatever happens. I can feel whatever feelings come up. I don't want to die, but I've accepted that I'm doing everything I can and if my number is up, then it's up. When the time comes, I can see myself going peacefully, knowing that it is my time to go, and believing that where I go from here is the next great adventure. In the meantime, I am making the most of this borrowed time.

The late great John Lennon wrote a song called "Borrowed Time" (included on his last album) which was inspired by a sailing adventure he was on in the spring of 1980. He had been in a creative dry spell for five years and was feeling depressed and decided to shake up his life by sailing with a crew on a 42-foot sailboat from Newport, Rhode Island to Bermuda. Not long into the journey a severe, life-threatening storm with 20-foot waves and 65 mile-per-hour winds rendered everyone on board seasick...except John. He was an inexperienced sailor and felt terrified, but he was the only one who was well enough to sail the boat.

He recounted in a Playboy interview a few months after the incident: "So, I was there driving the boat for six hours, keeping it on course. I was smashed in the face by waves for six solid hours. A couple of the waves had me on my knees. I was just hanging on with my hands on the wheel – it's very powerful weather – and I was having the time of my life."

He went on to say, "Once I accepted the reality of the

situation, something greater than me took over and all of a sudden I lost my fear. I actually began to enjoy the experience and I started to shout out old sea shanties in the face of the storm, screaming at the thundering sky."

When he got to Bermuda he said, "I was so centered after the experience at sea that I was tuned in, or whatever, to the cosmos. And all these songs came!" He had stepped up to the challenge, faced his fear, faced death, and came through it invigorated, enlivened and inspired to write the beautiful songs for his Double Fantasy album, which eventually won the Grammy for album of the year.

After that incident John realized that he was living on borrowed time and said, "Come to think of it, that's what we all are doing, even though most of us don't like to face it." He was killed just 6 months after that great awakening and brilliant outpouring of creativity, but I imagine that those 6 months were richly imbued with vivid aliveness and appreciation for the fragility and preciousness of life. I know that's what I'm feeling about my life.

When someone as world-renowned as John Lennon dies at such an early age, it reminds us that this earth life is finite and while we're still here, let's go for it, let's prioritize, let's live fully. As John said, we are ALL living on borrowed time. It's all gravy.

Are you fully tasting and savoring the gravy? Are you creating seeming catastrophes that are actually blessings in disguise, enhancing the flavor of your life, making it more delicious, exciting and purposeful? Here's to a life fully lived and savored!

# 47

## CHICKENS IN PARADISE
(February, 2011)

I have made a big decision…I've decided to get a PET CT scan and find out what is happening with the cancer in my body, and answer the questions, "Is it still there? Is it spreading? Is it completely gone?" Up until now I haven't wanted to know (and doctors said there was nothing more they could do anyway). I've been reluctant to know because I'm aware that my attitude affects my health. I know that relaxing and imagining myself whole and healed, as I've been doing, turns on healing genes, and stress turns them off. I didn't want to risk stressing out and turning off the healing genes.

What is different now are a couple of things. For one, I've discovered an alternative treatment called Paw Paw that is said to heal cancer about 50% of the time. The data and testimonials are very encouraging for all stages and types of cancer, so if I do still have cancer, I have a plan. Also, it is just possible that a scan will show that the cancer is already completely gone. How cool would that be!

What else is different is that I no longer feel my attitude would plummet if I learned the cancer is still in me, at least not for long. I am willing to fully feel whatever waves of feelings come up and surf them back to solid ground where I remember I am loved, I am guided, I am watched over, and I am right where I'm supposed to be. One thing life has taught me is that my attitude creates heaven or hell and I am responsible for my attitude. As the saying goes, "Life is 10%

what happens to us and 90% how we respond to it."

Tom and I were recently considering a trip to the beautiful island of Kauaii where we could stay for free for seven days in a timeshare gifted to us by dear friends. I started researching the island and found out it is a lush garden paradise, AND it is overrun by feral chickens and roosters! Some people think they're funny little critters and aren't bothered by them, some even think they're beautiful; but others think that the constant cacophonous squawking and cockadoodle-dooing make it seem like little pointy-beaked devils have turned paradise into hell. It is all in the eyes and ears of the beholder. I am sensitive to noise and it would be a 'hell' of a challenge for me, but if I really wanted to I think I could reframe the little peckers into heavenly creatures! It all depends on what I choose to focus on.

It's like the story about the Cherokee grandfather who is telling his grandchild about two wolves inside him. I'd like to tell you my version of that story: A Grandfather says to his grandchild, "A fight is going on inside me between two chickens. One chicken is always…well…feeling kind of chicken—worried and squawking and nit picking about every little thing. The other chicken is strutting its stuff, singing with joy, feeling like one of God's beloved creatures, trusting that it won't be deep fried and become someone's dinner, knowing that even if that happened, it is an eternal being and life will go on in another form. This same fight is going on inside of everyone." His grandchild asked, "Which chicken will win, Grandfather?" The grandfather simply replied, "The one you feed."

Even though I can be a big chicken at times, I can also be a brave chick filled with hope and faith—that is the one I intend to feed. But if the fearful chicken in me starts squawking, I will just love it, pet its ruffled feathers, allowing it to be where it is, until it calms down and transforms into the faith-filled chick that knows I am safe, I am loved, and all is well no matter what happens.

I don't have much control over what happens in life but I do have control over how I choose to perceive and respond to it. I am ready to face what is happening in my body and will not chicken out on getting the PET scan; though I might squawk a little bit—it is a bit scary. But I know I can cockadoodle do this! If the scan shows there's no more cancer, I will crow about it from the rooftops! If there is cancer, I will continue my alternative healing regimen, adding Paw Paw to it, and if it works I will also crow about it for all to hear. If it doesn't work, well then, I will fly the coop when the time comes, moving on to the next great adventure!

Do you have two chickens fighting inside you? Which one are you feeding? They're both God's children. Give them a hug from me.

## 48

## HEALING REGIMEN AND RESOURCES
(February 17, 2011)

I have received the results of the PET CT scan I had on Friday. It showed that there was hypermetabolic activity only in the area where the tumor was, where the radiation treatment was focused. I'm very relieved that it is localized and hasn't spread. The conclusion of the scan reads as follows:

"Stable appearance to mild hypermetabolic activity about the rectum. This is a nonspecific finding and may represent minimal inflammatory change. However, the possibility of neoplastic disease cannot be entirely excluded."

The results are inconclusive and my oncologist said that only a biopsy would tell for sure (which is too invasive so I don't intend to get one). What lit up on the scan could be inflammation from the radiation treatment, or it could be that a bit of cancer still remains. I like that they used the words "stable" and "mild".

My plan is to continue to do what I've been doing, since it seems to be working. I'd like to share my healing regimen with you. According to my research, everything on the list has been shown to have anti-cancer, healing ability. I recently added to this regimen the potent anti-cancer herb called Paw Paw, which is the only known substance that kills multi-drug-resistant cancer cells.

This cancer journey has been a wake-up call AND a gift that has brought me to a place of more aliveness, greater awareness of the preciousness of life, deeper appreciation for my loved ones, being more on purpose, less fearful, more whole, and filled with gratitude for this eternal NOW moment. The journey continues!

## HEALING REGIMEN

<u>ANTI-CANCER DIET</u>

ANTI-ANGIOGENESIS FOODS (block formation of blood vessels that feed tumors):
*green tea*
*turmeric, garlic, nutmeg, lavender, ginger*
*milk thistle, D3, selenium*
*dark chocolate (yes!)*
*resveratrol*
*licorice*
*olive oil*
*tomato sauce*
*parsley, celery*
*kale, brussel sprouts, cauliflower, broccoli, bok choy*
*artichokes*
*maitake mushrooms*
*pumpkin*
*soy beans*
*cranberries, blackberries, strawberries, blueberries, raspberries, pineapple, plums, grapefruit, lemons*
~~~~~~
No sugar (sweeten with Stevia, or occasionally raw honey)
No dairy
Low hypoglycemic foods (no white flour, rice, pasta etc.)
Lots of greens (creating an alkaline state in the body)
Carrot juice
Omega 3 oil (flaxseed oil, walnuts, hemp oil)

## SUPPLEMENTS
Chinese herbs
Paw Paw
Garlic
Vitamin D3
Turmeric and Bromelain (NOW brand, my year-long pain stopped after I started taking 4 of these a day—the curcumin in turmeric fights cancer in numerous ways)
Ellagic acid (Meeker Red Raspberry Seed, 8 a day—good source is raspberrygold.com)
Low-Dose Naltrexone (prescription, can reduce tumors, read about it at http://www.lowdosenaltrexone.org/ldn_and_cancer.htm)

## PRACTICES
*Generate Positive Attitude/Faith/Trust*
Read uplifting books
Visualize healing
Scripting (start the day writing or speaking how I want it to be as if it were already so, such as "Today I feel healthy, strong, and vibrantly alive.")

*Reduce Stress*
Simplify my life
Become present in the moment
Deep abdominal breathing
Meditation
Lots of laughter
Lots of hugs
Love – activating the healing energy of love by focusing on my heart, breathing through my heart, feeling loved and loving

*Energy Work*
Reiki
Qigong

*Exercise (reduces stress and oxygenates the body)*
Dancing
Gentle bouncing activates lymphatic system
Walking in sunshine, nature

*Emotional Release*
Fully feel, face and embrace my feelings
EFT (tapping on meridian points to help release fears, stress.
See Chapter 49 for tapping instructions)

*Attitude Adjustment*
Accept that it is what it is
Fully receive the learning and lessons
Affirm life purpose – Recommit to life and do what I love
Receive guidance from Conscious Cancer Coach, Melanie
Brown (http://consciouscancerjourney.com/)

ANTI-CANCER BOOKS
*Outsmart Your Cancer – Alternative Non-Toxic Treatments that Work* by Tanya Harter Pierce

*Cancer-Free – Your Guide to Gentle, Non-Toxic Healing* by Bill Henderson

*Anti Cancer – A New Way of Life* by David Servan-Shreiber

*Embrace, Release, Heal* by Leigh Fortson

*Healing Cancer Peacefully* by Nancy Offenhauser

*The Complete Cancer Cleanse* by Cherie Calbom, John Calbom, Michael Mahaffey

INSPIRATIONAL BOOKS
*A Thousand Names for Joy – Living in Harmony with the Way Things Are* by Byron Katie

*No Death, No Fear – Comforting Wisdom for Life* by Thich Nhat Hanh

*Miracles Every Day – The Story of One Physician's Inspiring Faith and the Healing Power of Prayer* by Maura Poston Zagrans

*The Nature of Personal Reality* by Jane Roberts

*The Spontaneous Healing of Belief* by Gregg Braden

*Journey of Souls – Case Studies of Life Between Lives* by Michael Newton

*Now That I Have Cancer I Am Whole – Reflections on Life and Healing for Cancer Patients and Those Who Love Them* by John Robert McFarland

*The Intention Experiment – Using Your Thoughts to Change Your Life and World* by Lynne McTaggert

*Living Well With Pain & Illness – The Mindful Way to Free Yourself from Suffering* by Vidyamala Burchko

*Spontaneous Healing* by Dr. Andrew Weil

*When Things Fall Apart: Heart Advice for Difficult Times* by Pema Chodron

*The Power of Now: A Guide to Spiritual Enlightenment* by Eckhart Tolle

*Healing With Love: A Breakthrough Mind/Body Medical Program for Healing Yourself and Others* by Dr. Leonard Laskow

**49**

# REALLY, TRULY, DEEPLY
# FREE AND CLEAR
(March 1, 2011)


Rumi said, "Your task is not to seek for love, but merely to seek and find all the barriers within yourself that you have built against it." Our natural state is love, health and wholeness. With cancer cells possibly still remaining in my body (according to my recent PET scan), I am on a full-scale mission to clear, clean and purify myself physically and emotionally, removing the barriers that keep me from love, health and wholeness.

Physically I have been doing a healing regimen that deeply cleans and clears my body (described in Chapter 48). I am also doing deep clearing and cleaning on an emotional level and I want to share with you three powerful tools I've combined for optimal inner cleansing.

One is called Ho'oponopono, an ancient Hawaiian healing tradition (ho'o means cause and ponopono means perfection). It's modern form is taught by Dr. Hew Len, who is famous for having healed an entire ward of criminally insane people at Hawaii State Hospital in the 1980's, without therapy, simply by doing Ho'oponopono on himself.

Its basic premise is that everything in our life is a projection—just like in a dream, it is all an aspect of ourselves. Whatever shows up in our life is our memories and old programming replaying 'out there', showing us where we are blocked from our true divine self. The way to clear these programs and return to our pure essence state is to say these words over and over until we are clear, "I love you. I'm sorry. Please forgive me. Thank you."

Conflict "out there" is cleared "in here", and once clear we are in union with the divine. The beauty part is that in that clear, higher vibrational state we attract miracles. That state can be maintained by repeatedly saying to ourselves throughout the day, "I love you" and "Thank you". Doing this on a daily basis aligns us with a state of grace place where life unfolds easefully and magically. That's where I want to live!

I have found that doing EFT while doing Ho'oponopono makes it even more powerful. EFT stands for Emotional Freedom Technique, an extremely effective healing method that involves tapping on specific meridian points to clear negative beliefs, feelings and programs from our body and bring in new desired beliefs (see the end of this chapter for EFT instructions). When you add to that some deep, slow breaths with long out-breaths, it further clears away the charge, since our reactive programming is locked in by shallow breaths and is set free by deep, full breaths.

I recently had an opportunity to put these three clearing superpowers to the test. I was having a conflict with someone in my life that set my two inner chickens to fighting. One chicken, Chicken Little, felt victimized, with feathers ruffled, lots of plaintive squawking, and she wanted to fly the coop. The other chicken, my glorious Warrioress Chicken Supreme, wanted to fly with the eagles and thus kept bringing me back to the awareness, "If it's in your life, it's in you. Now is an opportunity to clear and heal this inside yourself."

While one part of me was having a furious uprising, the other was having a spiritual "upwising" (as Swamibeyondananda would say). As I witnessed myself preparing for a defensive battle, I thought, "Since it's my creation, why not prepare for peace—instead of imagining a battle ahead, I can imagine peace."

Realizing the other person was mirroring a wounded part of myself, I loved that wounded part in me. Whenever I felt the furious wet-hen uprising within, I'd repeat the words, "I love you. I'm sorry. Please forgive me. Thank you." I added the meridian tapping and deep, slow breaths and the result was a peaceful resolution of the conflict. It proves the saying, "My how you've changed since I've changed." When I shift inside, my world shifts outside. I can choose love and peace, and clear whatever gets in the way of that with Ho'oponopono, meridian tapping, and deep slow breaths.

There's a wonderful story about Nelson Mandela (as told in the book *Buddha's Brain*) who was imprisoned for 27 years. His greatest despair was that he would lose contact with loved ones, as he was only allowed to receive letters from them about every 6 months. He didn't want to live without loving connections, so he decided he was going to bring love to the guards. By loving them it was hard for them to treat him harshly, therefore guards were frequently replaced; but he would simply love the new ones too. Despite the harshness of prison and hard labor, he chose to focus on love and that's what he experienced. Though he was in prison, he was FREE of hatred and anger.

These three tools, Ho'oponopono, tapping, and deep slow breaths, help to release old programming and clear away the barriers to love, healing and wholeness. This results in miracles and major life shifts. Toward that end, I am doing the Ho'oponopono with my body and the cancer; I'm tapping and breathing and saying, "I love you. I'm sorry. Please forgive me. Thank you." As I continue to do this healing work I'm hoping that down the road the results of my next PET scan will declare, "You are clean! You are free of cancer!"

Maybe even more important to me would be if one day I were able to declare that I am emotionally "free of charge", having successfully cleared away all my hot buttons. That is the ultimate freedom! What a monumental accomplishment that would be! Then I would be easefully, peacefully residing in the state of grace place, in the divine, in the field "out beyond right doing and wrong doing" that Rumi talks about. At the end of my life I want my epitaph to read, "Really, truly, deeply free at last!"

How about you? Do you have barriers within that are keeping you from love, health and wholeness? It's all an inside job. You can LOVE, TAP and BREATHE your way through those barriers and celebrate becoming free and clear and open to miracles!


EFT TAPPING INSTRUCTIONS:
Connect with and feel the issue you want to work on.
The tapping is 5-7 times per point.
Just do one side of the body.
Use two fingers to tap.
Choose a number from 1-10, gauging the intensity of the issue. Do several sequences, and at the beginning of each one decide what the number is. It will usually go down considerably as you repeat the cycles.
You can use the Ho'oponopono words on the sequence: "I love you. I'm sorry. Please forgive me. Thank you," using one phrase per tapping point. Or, you can choose a specific issue (see example given below).


THE SEQUENCE
This first tapping area is done only at the beginning:
TAP on side of hand, between base of pinky finger and wrist and repeat three times:
"Even though…(state the issue, example: "I feel scared about cancer.")…I deeply and completely accept myself."

TAP Top of head – summarize issue in a few words (such as "this fear").

Continue to repeat issue throughout the tapping sequence.

TAP Inner eyebrow

TAP Outer eyebrow

TAP Under eye, directly under pupil

TAP Under nose, in the little crevice

TAP Chin, in the depression between lip and chin

TAP Collar bone, just below knob of collarbone

TAP Under Arm, six inches below arm pit

Go back to head and repeat sequence

Eventually as your number decreases, you can add positive words about what it is you're wanting and beginning to feel. Such as: "Feeling calmer." "Feeling peaceful." "Feeling safe now." Etc.

This is a very simplified, bare-bones description.

For a free tapping e-book with more information, go to: http://www.thetappingsolution.com/

## 50

## PRONOIA INSTEAD OF PARANOIA
(March 21, 2011)

This is one freakin' scary, exciting, dramatic, shaking, shift-inducing ride we are all on together on planet earth! In light of the recent earthquake and tsunami disaster in Japan, and the continuing possible peril from a nuclear meltdown, it brings up the question: Is the universe friendly or is it fiendish? I vote for friendly, because while many of us when faced with our vulnerability on this precarious planet are scared to death, many more are scared to life! We are shakened and awakened and motivated to turn to the only thing that has permanence...the ultimate safety of an eternal, all-loving, omnipotent higher power.

That has been my experience with my own inner earthquake/bodyquake called cancer. It's caused me to feel, as writer John Perry Barlow wrote, "Pronoia—the suspicion that the Universe is a conspiracy on your behalf." I have come to believe that ALL of life is benevolently designed to wake us up to love, to our true self, and our higher purpose. Rob Brezsny writes in his book *Pronoia is the Antidote for Paranoia,* "No matter how upside down it all may appear, we will have no fear, because we know this big secret: All of creation is conspiring to shower us with blessings. Life is crazily in love with us – brazenly and innocently in love with us. The universe always gives us exactly what we need, exactly when we need it."

Be it earthquakes or cancer or any of the innumerable catastrophes that can befall vulnerable humans, when shit happens it spurs shift to happen and turns it into gold. The entire planet literally shifted on its axis from this powerful 9.0 quake…and many people have shifted as a result into more love, compassion, empathy, generosity, purposefulness, presence, and the awareness that we are all connected.

Some of the exquisite beauty that has arisen from this terrible tragedy is evidenced in many of the heart-warming, soul-stirring stories being reported. For example:

A news crew shot footage of two muddy, disheveled dogs in the middle of scattered rubble. One dog was anxiously hovering over the other dog, who was lying beside him, immobile. The anxious dog moved towards the camera crew and then back to his stricken buddy. He sat close beside him, putting his paw on his pals head, as if to say, "Please help my friend." Both dogs were rescued and are doing well.

There's an amazing story about an 83-year-old woman outrunning the tsunami on her bicycle! And there's the miracle of a four-month-old baby girl who was found buried in rubble for three days after having been swept from her parents arms when the terrible wave hit their home. She was reunited with her overjoyed parents unharmed. No one knows how it was she didn't drown.

More gold from this tragedy is the outpouring of love and compassion from all over the world. Even China, a long-time adversary of Japan, has reached out with rescue teams and millions of dollars in aid. Studies have found that such acts of compassion benefit the receiver AND the giver— for all involved it creates feel-good oxytocin, stimulates the immune system, and enhances feelings of serenity and fellowship. Compassion raises our vibration to a higher level of ourselves.

Another inspiring story is of the workers who are staying behind at the nuclear plant to try and avert a meltdown. They are true heroes, putting the good of others ahead of themselves. It's possible that on the *soul level* the courageous people of Japan who lost loved ones or their own lives may have volunteered for this great mission...a mega heroes journey, helping to catalyze immense compassion in the world, reminding us all of the fragility and impermanence of earth and body, and the all-embracing permanence of spirit, as well as reminding us to cherish our life and those we love.

When I first learned that my cancer had returned and my chances of survival were slim and that most probably great pain and suffering was ahead, there were times when I just wanted to check out of Hotel Earth. "Get me out of here!" I hoped that a bolt of lightening or a heart attack would strike and spare me from the ordeal ahead. I wanted to bypass the terrible fear, pain, and suffering. But instead I turned towards spirit and asked for help and guidance and it came. Fear became faith, paranoia became pronoia, and I was led to finding precious gold amidst the rubble.

In times of crisis our frightened ego may feel like the sky is falling, yet our awakened spirit remembers, "I am the sky." Life can seem like a terrible trial, but if you move the 'i' forward in the word trial it becomes 'trail', a trail that leads us Home, to spirit, light, love, and more aliveness. This is all part of the divine plan of a friendly universe that wants only to awaken us.

Is your universe friendly or fiendish, *pro*noiac or paranoiac? Do you have any personal disasters shaking your world right now? From my perspective it's just the universe shaking and waking you to your magnificent Big Soul Self. "All of creation is conspiring to shower you with blessings" no matter how it may appear.

# 51

## IT'S ABOUT LOVE!

(April 3, 2011)

I was deeply impressed years ago by a story actress Shirley Maclaine told about her father, a gruff, curmudgeonly old man, who was on his deathbed. He was drifting in and out of consciousness, back and forth between this world and the next, when suddenly he woke up, his eyes opened wide, and in a eureka moment he exclaimed, "I get it—it's about love! It's all about love!"

I get it now too. It's one of the most rousing wake-up calls I've received from my cancer adventure. I am galvanized to use what time I have left in this earth suit to learn to love more, to open my heart, loving all my unloved body parts, loving my feelings, loving this precious moment, loving others, loving life—I have woken up to the realization that it's all about love!

Love is a powerful energy. I believe that the energy of love raises our vibration and all that is not love falls away. I am therefore very motivated to actively cultivate the healing energy of love. Ever since my Big C journey began, I have been doing a practice when I wake up in the morning of imagining love energy flowing into my head from above, down to my heart and from my heart down my arms into my hands. I place my hands over my wounded lower region for several minutes while love flows through my hands into that area of my body. That could be one of the reasons I'm healing. I know that my whole being relaxes and feels uplifted when I do that.

I'm reminded of The Institute of HeartMath's simple formula for cultivating the energy of love and harmony in ourselves: First, focus on your heart. Then breathe through your heart. Next imagine someone or something that evokes the feeling of love in you. I put this formula to the test recently when I was having trouble falling asleep. I started to focus on my heart, breathing through my heart, imagining warm, pink, shimmering light in my heart, and feeling love and gratitude for Tom lying beside me. My monkey mind settled down and sweet sleep finally came! I do that every night now. I fall asleep in love.

We don't need to have a partner to focus our love on; we can love anything, and the energy of love will be activated. Nearly every day I go on "I love" walks. As I walk, I love the yellow flowers, I love the mountains, I love the blue sky, I love the little scurrying lizards. Some days I need to love myself for not feeling very loving—I love my curmudgeon self. Love is love, it doesn't matter what we love, all that matters is that we love.

Dis-ease and challenges can be a great form of resistance training for building our love muscles. Last October when I was feeling lousy from the effects of chemo and radiation and thought my days were numbered, to my surprise I decided to join a woman's group. I've never been a 'group' person. I have wonderful, loving, one-on-one relationships, but being in a group sometimes rattles my defenses about criticism and feeling controlled. It can reactivate old family dynamics— my rebel imagines opposition and braces for a struggle, and therefore, that's exactly what I create. I wondered, "What the heck am I doing in a woman's group?"

Now I get it…it's about love! My trouper soul says, "Oh goody, let's use being in this group as a probe to bring up our 'stuff' so that we can exercise the act of choosing love. Let's learn and grow as much as we can while we can." (I love my trouper soul!) In my group I'm learning to shift my focus from my head, where the battle is taking place, to my heart, where peace and love prevail. As each woman speaks, I imagine a line of light from my heart to hers. When my critical mind starts to take over again, I shift my focus back to my heart. I end up feeling all warm and fuzzy, floating in a sea of oxytocin (our inner love potion). Through this filter of love I see the beauty of each woman, including myself, and I experience loving kindness from and towards these women.

I love sending out my newsletter but sometimes it brings up my fears of criticism, rejection, and the fear of making a mistake. Several newsletters ago I did make a mistake. I forgot to do the blind copy for the e-mail addresses and sent it out with all of them exposed. I cringed. "Dang! I can't believe I did that!" Then I remembered, "It's about love. This is an opportunity to reprogram this fear and choose love. Instead of imagining criticism and rejection, I can imagine love." I visualized the e-mail list forming the shape of a heart, and I sent love to the list as a whole, and imagined love coming back to me. I do that each time now when I send out a new newsletter. It's all part of my training to love and feel loved.

What the world needs now is love, sweet love. It has been a difficult few weeks for me and for many people that I know. I think the disaster in Japan has unsettled people, triggering pain and stirring old internal debris. Many people are having their own personal inner earthquakes, tsunamis and meltdowns. I know that's true for me. The other day there was an exquisite sunset and my friend Joy said, "Look, it's an angel." Contrasted vividly against the aqua blue sky was a large, bright, coral pink cloud that looked like an angel looking down on us. It was a beautiful, timely reminder to me that we are loved and watched over.

I am building my home in love. It is the energy I want to cultivate and live in. I used to live in fear and visit love, but now, more and more, I live in love and occasionally visit fear. Love is becoming my home base…though I can always count on resistance training to present itself so that I can keep strengthening my love muscles. Sometimes it takes calamities and discord to wake us up to love. But it doesn't have to…love is a moment-to-moment choice. Right now, I choose love.

How about you? Are you choosing love in this moment? It is our true home—home is where the heart is.

# 52

## PERFECTLY IMPERFECT
(May 14, 2011)

Wabi Sabi (wah-bee sah-bee) is a Japanese concept of life and art in which beauty is found in things that are weathered, asymmetrical, incomplete, imperfect and impermanent. As I age, my body is becoming all of the above! Therefore, Wabi Sabi has become my new kemo sahbee (faithful friend). I'm learning to see myself as a work of art, not in spite of my flaws, but BECAUSE of them. What a concept!

I've had a head start with this Wabi Sabi way of seeing myself—over the years I've been learning to face my emotional flaws and accept myself as perfectly imperfect. I was motivated to do this by a painful sense of shame and a belief that I was fundamentally flawed and needed to be perfect in order to be loved. The quest for perfection put a cork in my aliveness that eventually caused me to crack under the pressure. This set me on a new quest to learn to love myself AS IS, warts and all. I am still on that journey. I am learning to love my imperfect self.

One of my favorite quotes that has helped me in reframing my flawed self is Ashleigh Brilliant's epigram, "I may not be perfect, but parts of me are excellent!" I've said this to myself many times throughout the years and it's always made me feel better about myself. Now, in the spirit of Wabi Sabi, I tell myself, "I may not be perfect, but my imperfections make me unique and beautiful!" Krishnamurti has said that our souls are from the same paper but what makes us unique is the creases formed in the paper from all the folding and unfolding of our life experience.

This Wabi Sabi perspective is helping me face and embrace my body upheavals of the last several years. Despite my careful attempts to remain perfectly in tact, Bell's palsy set my face permanently askew, gum disease ate away at my jawbone, cataracts clouded my eyes, an appendectomy removed my ruptured appendix, and cancer devoured my uterus, (not to mention the addition of wrinkles and gray hair, oy!).

I have had to let go of my attachment to things being perfect. I've chosen instead to see and accept the beauty of this cracked, weathered vessel that I've become. A little boy said to his grandmother, "Oh Gramma, you have such beautiful designs on your face." I'm learning to see myself the way that little boy sees his grandmother.

There is great liberation in perceiving ourselves as beautiful, not in spite of our flaws, but because of them. It is heartening to see ourselves as not broken, but instead broken open—all the better to receive the abundant light and love that surrounds us. Leonard Cohen echoes this sentiment in his song, Anthem:

*Ring the bells that still can ring*
*Forget your perfect offering*
*There is a crack in everything*
*That's how the light gets in.*

Finally I'd like to leave you with the quintessential Wabi Sabi story of the Cracked Pot: Everyday a waterbearer carried two pots balanced on a yoke across his shoulders to his master's house. One of the pots was cracked and leaked water all the way there. This made the pot very sad. "I'm so imperfect. Why do you keep me?" The waterbearer answered, "I planted flowers along your side of the path and the water you spill nourishes those flowers. Because of you, the beautiful flowers that grow there have brought great joy to my master. Your flaws bring joy and beauty."

The story we tell ourselves about our lives is always our choice. It can be a sob story, or a Wabi Sabi story. We can choose to see ourselves as a crackpot or as a cracked pot watering flowers on our life path. I am choosing to see my life as a perfect work of art, cracks and all!

What's your Wabi Sabi story? Can you see how your flaws, imperfections, and challenges have made your life a beautiful work of art?

## 53

# OXYTOCIN, THE CUDDLE CURE
(May 29, 2011)

I've been getting high on the hug drug, the cuddle cure, the happy hormone called oxytocin. This week I've had an upsurge of this potent love potion since I found a crying, starving, trembling, abandoned feral kitten about 6 weeks old living under the bushes near my house. Seeing him so tiny and helpless and all alone in the world made my heart melt and I was aflood with oxytocin. He wouldn't let me near him, but fueled by this powerful 'tend and befriend' hormone, I was determined to help him.

Off and on over the course of three days I sat with him, absorbed in a meditative stillness, talking to him sweetly, patiently luring him nearer to me by moving the food I brought him closer and closer. Eventually, he came up to me, brushed his head against my hand and started purring! I was beside myself with oxytocin momma love!

I took him home with me and we have been passionately engaged in cuddle storms of mutual love! What a feeling! It's no wonder they call it the happy hormone. I feel this same feeling for my other cats as well—I am awash in warm fuzzy feelings for my warm fuzzy felines! That includes my Tom cat, my husband Tom, the warm fuzzy fella I cuddle with every day.

I love oxytocin! It is a natural high that creates feelings of peace, calm, wellbeing, compassion, trust, and altruism. Starting from infancy with the mother-child connection, it is the glue that bonds us to loved ones and makes them appear more appealing to us. Just thinking about people we love evokes this love hormone (which is produced in our brain AND our hearts).

Studies have found that when we have high levels of oxytocin in our system, we are like a tuning fork and those around us start resonating with our peaceful vibe and their oxytocin levels increase as well. That's why we like to be around loving people, because we feel more loving in their presence. Oxytocin is contagious!

It is often called the 'cuddle cure' because it has tremendous health benefits, which include lowering our blood pressure, raising our pain threshold, boosting our immune system and reducing stress (the precursor and aggravator of most illnesses). Due to Oxytocin, people with pets often heal from illness more quickly, and people in cancer support groups have a tendency to live longer—tend and befriend equals mend.

For that reason, the cuddle cure is a big part of my healing regimen. Stress exacerbates cancer by turning off healing genes, while love and serenity turn on healing genes. Therefore, I'm motivated to steep myself like a tea bag in the healing elixir of oxytocin as often as I can!

There are many ways to stimulate oxytocin production. It is activated in response to touch, massage, sex, kisses, appreciation, gratitude, loving relationships, compassion, and caring for others. Hugging for at least 20 seconds increases oxytocin. Even just visualizing hugging others activates it. You can give imaginary hugs to people all day long, people you don't even know, and you will reap the benefits. I've been practicing sending love from my heart to the heart of others, and I am flooded with the warm, peaceful love energy that I'm sending.

Self-compassion is another way to generate oxytocin. Lady Gaga, a champion of self-love, practices self-compassion for five minutes each morning. Imagine the feel-good fun of having a verbal cuddle fest with yourself every day!

Meditation is a powerful stimulator of this healing hormone. Years ago, when I lived alone, I meditated each morning and was blissfully bathed in oxytocin. I got high on the feeling of being deeply connected and loved by the higher energy that held me in a warm spiritual hug. When I began living with Tom I didn't meditate as much; but now, ever since my cancer diagnosis, I am back to deeply connecting and cuddling with spirit on a regular basis.

When I hold my new little bitty kitty and reassure him that he is loved and cared for and his hard-knock life is a thing of the past, I imagine that my higher power is reassuring me in the same way. I am comforted in the faith that my higher self is watching over me, flooding me with love, telling me, "You are safe, you are loved, all is well, you have found your way to a friendly place." My higher self and I luxuriate in rapturous oxytocin love fests! What a feeling! Can you hear me purring?

Have you been getting high on the love drug, oxytocin? Are there ways that you can increase this powerful love potion in your life even more? I'm sending you a warm hug and sharing some of my 'stash' with you!

## 54

# CALLING ON FIERCENESS
(June 12, 2011)

Worry thoughts about the state of my health have been nipping at my heels of late—much like my new kitten that I rescued (and named Wabi), who is literally nipping at my heels, determinedly insisting on sinking his teeth and claws into life and into me! He is a persistent little whirling cactus! His new big bro Bo (our other cat) is ten times his size and could eat him for breakfast, but to Wabi, he is a pony to mount and ride and roll around on and play with. Bo swats Wabi away but he relentlessly bounds back. He is fearless! And fierce! And he wants to PLAY!

He is my current model for determination and unabashed living! That's the spirit that helped this little one-pounder survive in the wilds all by himself for days, until a blonde giant (moi) strolled by and he cried out to me with a loud, bellowing meow. With that volume of voice I expected a huge cat, but instead a tiny ball of fur appeared from under the bushes, with his urgent, demanding, attention-commanding MEOW!!!

I need that kind of fierceness now. The universe is demanding of me, "Be HERE now", NOT in the feared, imagined future. Trying to bring myself back to the present moment once fear thoughts have taken over can feel as if I'm herding cats. My fears are like feral cats who see danger everywhere, even though love and aid is being offered. When my new kitten chose to trust the love that was offered, he hit the lotto and is now- nestled in the lap of luxury. He is reminding me to be brave and trust like he did.

To help me come back to trust, I've been reciting in my mind the line from the poem Desiderata, that says, "Whether or not it is clear to you, no doubt the universe is unfolding as it should." I take a deep breath of relief with that. As someone who has come to the planet to learn and grow and evolve my consciousness, I can see how my soul might have chosen cancer in order to galvanize me to get on with that work. I distinctly remember a time just before my initial diagnosis when I was lying on the couch watching television, feeling lazy and bored, and I had the thought, "What am I doing here? I'm frittering away my time."

I'm not frittering my time away anymore! With fierce determination, ever since my cancer diagnosis, I've been focused on transforming my hell-raising fears into heaven-raising faith. When I get off track, like I occasionally do, I always come back to my life-affirming practices of focusing on my heart, meditating, gratitude, trust, acceptance, deep breathing, walking in nature, and dancing. "I get up. I walk. I fall down. Meanwhile, I keep dancing."-(Rabbi Hillel) That brings me back to an expansive place where I feel like a child at play with colored balls, or, better yet, a kitten at play with EVERYTHING!

We are all gods with amnesia, waking up to who we truly are. Sometimes the universe sends us things to help remind us…like cancer and kittens. When I think about the challenges we souls take on here on planet earth, I am in awe of our courage and spirit. I agree with Rumi who said, "When you see your beauty, you will become your own idol."

How about you? Has life been calling on your fierce persistence and determination to meet, greet, and defeat the challenges in your life?

## 55

# FROM HYPER-VIGILANCE TO
# HIGHER VIGILANCE
(June 27, 2011)

I sometimes call my new kitten Buddha-Pest because at times he has the serenity of a Buddha, but at other times he is a pest—nipping, biting, and digging his claws into anything that moves! This is much like my mind, which at times rests in a sublime state of peace and acceptance, and at other times pesters me with gnawing, clawing fear thoughts, like, "What's that ache? What's that twinge? Why am I so tired? Could it be the cancer is back!?"

I wish I could rest in a Buddha-full state of serenity all the time, but my mind is ever alert for danger. That's what the lower reptilian brain does—its prime directive is survival and avoiding harm. For that reason, according to Rick Hanson, author of the book *Buddha's Brain: The Practical Neuroscience of Happiness, Love, and Wisdom*, painful experiences are much more easily and deeply imprinted in our brains than pleasurable ones. He explains that there is "an innate negativity bias of the brain, whose unfortunate default setting is to be Velcro for negative experiences but Teflon for positive ones."

Here's an example: A few weeks ago I saw a three-foot snake on the nature path behind my house. It was patiently poised beside a gopher hole, so I'm assuming it was a gopher snake. Nevertheless, it was a SNAKE! And it was BIG! I haven't been back there since...until today. I walked along the path, vigilantly scanning for snakes, seeing twigs, and even shadows of branches, as snakes. Even though I was surrounded by beautiful nature, all I could envision was snakes! I sadly realized, "Every time I walk here now I will be looking for snakes." The same is true with cancer...with each minor ache and pain and fatigue, my mind leaps to cancer.

Buddhists call this "the pain of pain"—the initial pain is unavoidable, but the reaction to that pain, the fear and resistance to it, is self-inflicted. The challenge is to get free of the pain of pain, to let go of negative reactions, because those reactions and perceptions are what cause the greatest suffering.

I want to walk along life's path and see the beautiful flowers, the blue sky, the mountains, instead of imagining twigs as snakes and twinges as cancer. I want to be *higher*-vigilant instead of hyper-vigilant—to see life from the higher perspective of my soul, where I remember that I am an eternal being, where I know that cancer is my great teacher, life enhancer, and burr under my saddle that woke me up and keeps me awake!

Fortunately, the higher brain has neuroplasticity, which is the ability to learn from experience and imprint the positive new learning. But in order for this to happen, research shows that the new belief and feeling needs to be repeated many, many times. Fear is an easy neural pathway to go down. Faith needs to be repeated over and over again. Therefore, whenever fear appears, I higher-vigilantly remind myself, "What's the truth? The truth is that right now I am safe. Right now all is well. Right now is all there is." I breathe a big, deep breath, really feeling and letting in this belief.

Rick Hansen says we need to hold the desired thought and feeling for about 30 seconds so that it can imprint in our memory. We need to bathe in it for a bit and feel it fully. He says, "The longer that something is held in awareness and the more emotionally stimulating it is, the more neurons that fire and thus wire together. The more you get your neurons firing about positive facts, the more they'll be wiring up positive neural structures."

I am passionately intent on firing and wiring beautiful, Buddha-full neural pathways in my brain—pathways where a snake is just a snake, simply another of God's creatures, and a twinge is just twinge, reminding me to breathe and turn from hyper-vigilance to higher-vigilance, and cancer is just a kick in the can, waking me up to my true self, my Big Ass Soul Self.

Being in a state of higher vigilance helps me put the 'can' in cancer, as in I *can* do this, I *can* learn and grow from this, I *can* remember that I am watched over, loved and guided, I *can* be present with whatever happens, fully, deeply present. I'm feeling all fired up now! I'm going to go dance a rousing rendition of the *cancan* to help fire and wire this feeling!

Is your mind a Buddha-pest, serene at times but pestering you with habitual, hyper-vigilant worry thoughts? I invite you to shift into higher-vigilance and fire and wire up some new, positive, life-enhancing neural pathways. Yes you can can!

## 56

## NO HURRY, NO WORRY
(August 13, 2011)

Years ago I saw a movie in which a busy, stressed-out woman was diagnosed with terminal cancer and, understandably, she was terrified. She started working with a Chinese doctor who taught her the healing power of relaxation and told her to repeat the mantra, "No hurry, no worry." She said those words often and followed his healing regimen and was eventually cured! Those words have stayed with me over the years and I often say them to myself whenever I feel stressed. "No hurry, no worry." Or, as my teenage niece says, "Chillax!"

There's a direct correlation between stress and illness, especially cancer. We all have cancer cells in our bodies and a strong immune system is what keeps them from multiplying. However, stress suppresses the immune system, and in some people this allows cancer to grow out of control. Stress also creates an acidic condition in the body, which cancer thrives on. In addition, stress creates inflammation, another dangerous breeding ground for cancer and other illnesses.

When I think about what probably most contributed to my having cancer, the answer is stress. Many years ago I was aware of how much tension I had in my body—I noticed a habitual clenching, particularly in my stomach and pelvic area. I had the thought, "If I ever have health problems, this is where it will be." Sure enough, three years ago all hell broke loose down there, starting with a ruptured, necrotic, gangrenous appendix, the worst my doctor had ever seen, followed by the discovery of uterine cancer, and, finally, recurring uterine cancer.

Since stress turns off my immune system, in order to heal I know I need to relax. I can hear a frantic part of me imploring, "RELAX OR DIE!" But it's hard to relax with a cancer diagnosis; while tension is a precursor of cancer, it is also a natural reaction to it once you have it. Therefore, I am diligently committed to cultivating a relaxing path of "No hurry, no worry", which includes meditation, exercise, visualization, and trusting that I am loved and guided and right where I'm supposed to be.

Lately, I've added a new refrain, "Viva La Vagus!," in celebration of the amazing vagus nerve. (I've been singing the Elvis song, Viva Las Vegas, in my head all day!) I've recently learned that the vagus nerve activates the immune system, and deep, slow, abdominal breaths activate the vagus nerve.

I was alerted to this when my brilliant scientist friend, Peggy LaCerra, wrote on Facebook, "When people are panicked because of an illness, I tell them to simply take 10 VERY DEEP breaths repeatedly throughout the day because, when we breath deeply, the diaphragm drops to the bottom of the thoracic cavity. The vagus nerve, the main 'neural cable' of the parasympathetic system, runs through the diaphragm muscle. When the diaphragm drops down and then rises and drops down and rises repeatedly, it stimulates the vagus nerve and initiates a shift back to a parasympathetic state." The parasympathetic state triggers a relaxation response and activates the immune system, helping our bodies heal, repair, and renew.

I've since been researching the vagus nerve and found that taking the deep, slow, abdominal breaths that trigger it promotes healing in numerous ways: it oxygenates the body (cancer hates oxygen), creates alkalinity in the body (cancer is said to flourish in acidity and wither in alkalinity), helps control obesity (which is another risk factor for cancer and other illnesses), reduces inflammation, makes our lymphatic system work better, improves memory, fights depression, lowers blood pressure, enhances brain and heart activity, purifies our blood, aids digestion, rejuvenates our skin, and reduces pain. Deep breathing delivers a wealth of health benefits! And it's completely FREE! I just need to remember to do it!

The healing power of breath is not news to me. After all, my e-mail address of the last ten years has been JanBreathe, because I wanted to remind myself to breathe. I've also studied breath work with breath master Gay Hendricks, and learned well the importance of conscious breathing. Yet...I forget, I go unconscious and revert back to my old habitual shallow breath.

But now, knowing that the best chance I have of completely healing from this life-threatening illness is having a strong immune system, and knowing that deep breath triggers the vagus nerve which in turn triggers the immune system, I'm all about breathing deep, slow breaths all day, every day! I want to live, and, also, it feels good! What I'm finding as I'm focusing on deep breathing is that it energizes and enlivens me. When I'm fully breathing, I'm fully alive. When I'm shallow breathing, I'm shallowly alive. "He lives most life whoever breathes most air."-(Elizabeth Barrett Browning)

I can see where early in life I unconsciously adopted a life strategy to breathe shallowly as a way to blunt my feelings. The flaw in that strategy is that shallow breathing contributes to stress, tension, illness, anxiety, depression, and more things to feel fear about. Fully breathing is committing to being in my body and feeling my full aliveness, including being willing to feel all my feelings.

As I breathe deep, slow breaths throughout the day, I'm feeling invigorated and calm at the same time. Being a multitasker, when I can remember, I add a smile to my breathing, (stimulating healing endorphins), and say the words "I love you" (activating healing oxytocin). As an added bonus to all the health benefits, I'm finding that focusing on deep breathing is an instant portal to the present moment. That's the place I want to be.

"Breathing in, I calm body and mind. Breathing out, I smile. Dwelling in the present moment I know this is the only moment."-(Thich Nhat Hanh) I say a big YES to fully breathing, being fully alive, fully in my body, AND fully healed! I'll breathe to that!

Are you committed to fully breathing and being fully alive? No hurry, no worry—just take some deep, slow breaths and join me in a rousing chorus of "Viva La Vagus!" Here's to a stimulated immune system and a stimulating life!

# 57

## DANCING IN THE RAIN
(August 22, 2011)

"Life isn't about waiting for the storm to pass…it's about learning to dance in the rain."-(Unknown)

Last week Tom and I went to the Summer Concert in the Park on the Santa Barbara waterfront and danced to the music of a Beatles tribute band. We moved our bodies in happy abandon in a sweet and sweaty crush of baby boomers and people of all ages. I was high on nostalgia, and at the same time, high on the present moment.

I felt that old thrill of excitement that was ignited all those years ago in the teenage me listening to my first Beatles songs, a thrill that shot through me like electricity, like a defibrillator jumpstarting my heart and my life. "Shake it up baby now, twist and shout!" It all came back. I loved the Beatles and that exciting time in my life, a time of rebirth into a new version of myself, a vibrant new burst of aliveness. I'm feeling that same bright-eyed aliveness now—a gift from cancer.

As I boogied to the Beatles music, my past and present weaved together. Back then it was the 60's…and now I'm IN my 60's! I flashed back in time, remembering The Travelons, the Beatles tribute band that was famous in the 1960's on the east coast, who I loved to dance to and was a bit of a groupie. I dated the drummer a few times, but was so shy I barely spoke—I needed to drink a beer or two to help me loosen up. "It's a good thing I look good," I thought back then.

On the ride to the Concert in the Park with Tom I caught a glimpse of myself in the car mirror, seeing the fine (and not so fine) lines sprinkled on my face, and thought, "It's a good thing Tom loves me for who I am, not how I look!" It's an even better thing that I finally feel beautiful INSIDE. That is a monumental life accomplishment for me! And I no longer need to drink a beer in order to feel uninhibited—I feel so much more comfortable in my skin now, wrinkled though it is.

Dancing to the beat of the Beatles songs, I felt like the teenage me of yesteryear. Yet in present time, there was Tom, holding me close, looking at me with happy, loving eyes, and I felt treasured, something the teenage me never felt. I did a mind-meld through time with my teenage self and told her, "Look who we end up with, this wonderful man! Look at where we live, this beautiful paradise on earth! Look at the wonderful friends we have, dancing with us!" Thinking about the whole of my life, I tell her, "What a journey you have ahead of you!" (Some say all time is simultaneous— if so my teenage self received a message of hope for the future).

I kept looking at Tom, his beautiful blue eyes, his luminous smile, his sweet soul, and I felt blown away that I ended up with such a fabulous man. My history with cancer adds poignancy to my happy moments with him. The uncertainty of it is always in the back of our minds. As we dance to a slow Beatles song, he presses his forehead against mine, looks into my eyes and says sweetly, "Don't go." "Okay, I'll stay" I say, smiling. But I can't help wondering if I'll be around for next summer's concerts in the park. I think about Beatles John and George, gone now. We just don't know what the future will bring. As John Lennon said, "We are all living on borrowed time."

Though I don't know what the future holds, I can allow myself to be fully held in this moment, in Tom's arms, in a feeling of celebration, savoring it all. Celebrating how far I've come and how much I've learned in this life. Celebrating the present moment, that I have arrived here at last! It has been a long journey to the Now, but I am Here Now a lot of the time—another gift of cancer.

At the dance, we talk to a friend who has a bum shoulder and other health issues requiring medical assistance. It is testing his fear of aging. But he tells us that he's decided to have fun with it. Instead of dreading going to the doctors, he has an attitude of celebrating and playing with it all. Ill health can make us feel like a failure, yet to feel joy in the midst of our challenges is a great success. As Emerson said, "To have played and laughed with enthusiasm, and sung with exultation—this is to have succeeded."

I'm here, facing my worst fears, feeling my feelings fully, AND playing and laughing with enthusiasm, singing along to old Beatle tunes with exultation! I may be here for many more years to come. Or not. I know that there's much I want to see and do. I have fully arrived at this earth party and I want to laugh and learn and play more! I'm reassured by Richard Bach's quote: "Here is the test to find whether your mission on earth is finished: If you're alive, it isn't." I'm alive, so it isn't!

In the Ram Dass book, *STILL HERE – Embracing Aging, Changing, and Dying*, despite a stroke that has incapacitated him in many ways, he sees how perfect it all is. It has helped him to even more fully *BE HERE NOW*, valuing this life, and knowing more deeply that he is not just a body, he is an eternal soul. That awareness helps make these earthly woes (or what Ram Dass calls 'bed of woeses') not so devastating. And, knowing that we will die makes life more precious. Because of that, I am not only still here, I am more HERE than I have ever been before! The 1960's were great, but I can honestly say that this life just keeps getting better and better!

If you could do a mind-meld through time with your teenage self, what would you say? Life is such a magical mystery tour; we can use all the love and encouragement we can get!

In closing, I'd like to share with you this celebratory song I wrote with my friend Nicola Gordon (sung to the tune, The Ants Going Marching One by One):

*There's nothing I have to do today – Hurrah, Hurrah!*
*There's nothing I have to do or say – Hurrah, Hurrah!*
*Just be in the NOW all the way*
*That's all I have to do today.*
*Breathe in, breathe out.*
*Sing and dance and play!*

## 58

# YOU ARE THE BOSS
# OF YOUR OWN REALITY
(September 10, 2011)

"You are the boss of your own reality." Those are the words in a handwritten letter sent to me years ago by Jane Roberts, who channeled the Seth books. I treasure that letter; but even more, I treasure that message. I am the boss of my own reality. I am creating and shaping the colorful play doh of my life with my feelings, beliefs, desires, expectations, and actions.

Some people call this "The Secret"...I call it "The Magic". It is the great love of my life that has thrilled, excited and motivated me for many years. It is the quantum paradigm shift from feeling like a hapless victim of circumstances to being an empowered creator of my life.

I was first introduced to this great love early in my life when I read, *Your Thoughts Can Change Your Life* by Donald Curtis. At that time I was a depressed teen who felt unlovable and feared that I'd always be alone. But that book set off fireworks in me! I was thrilled to know that if I changed my beliefs, I could change my reality. That began a long journey that took me clear across the country and across time where I eventually married the man of my dreams in the very church where Donald Curtis had been the minister!

The power of belief is not a new concept—Jesus talked about it more than 2000 years ago, saying: "If you can believe, all things are possible to him who believes." And, "I say to you, if you have faith as small as a mustard seed, you can say to this mountain, 'Move from here to there,' and it will move, and nothing will be impossible for you."

When I first met Tom, he lived in Minnesota and I lived in California. If the power of belief could move a mountain from here to there, I thought, surely it could move him from there to here! I got out my well-worn favorite Seth book, *The Nature of Personal Reality*, to help refresh and prime my manifesting skills...and, through passionate and dedicated application, I managed to MANifest this amazing man into my life! However, I found that first, in order for that to happen I needed to ferret out the beliefs that were unconsciously manifesting my being alone.

Once I faced those beliefs it was time to replace them. Here is Seth's magic formula that I faithfully followed: "For five minutes only, direct all of your attention toward what you want. Use visualization or verbal thought—whatever comes most naturally to you; but for that period do not concentrate upon any lacks, just upon your desire. In one way or another make one physical gesture or act that is in line with your belief or desire. Then forget about it." Doing this every day builds the vibrational energy of what you're wanting and magnetizes it to you.

My new relationship with Tom stirred up my pre-programmed emotional pain and defenses; but reading Seth's book kept reminding me that my beliefs and programming were the source of my pain, not Tom. I would ride out the emotional storms, and always come home to owning it as mine. Seth wrote: "Any feeling fully felt and experienced will always bring you back to love." It always did...the thunder was always followed by enlightening. As a result of my fierce tenacity to own that "I create my reality", I was rewarded with great love and respect from Tom, AND more importantly, from myself. I tell myself, "That's why God is paying me the big buck (that would be Tom, my big buck)!"

Through the power of belief, imagination and strong desire, anything is possible, anything can be changed and healed...even cancer. There are many stories of people using the power of visualization to heal themselves of cancer. My friend, nutritionist Dale Figtree, described to me a compelling account of how she healed a tumor overnight:

"I did a visualization of the cancer cells like black clumps of spiders on top of each other, inside a big volcano (so that they were contained.) Then at the top of the volcano surrounding it were hundreds of thousands of white blood cells as Knights in armor on white horses, carrying big lances. With a clash of symbols, they rode down into the volcano and slashed and punctured every single cancer cell, which in turn evaporated until there was nothing but pink healthy cells and a clear blue sky above. I really got deeply into it. Afterwards, I felt a serenity, and my fear was gone. I thought that was the gifting—until the next day when I went to be re-x-rayed — I was shocked to hear the tumor was gone!" (Dale writes more about how she cured herself of cancer in her book, *Beyond Cancer Treatment*.)

Now, once again I'm reading my Seth book to remind me that through the power of belief anything is possible. Every day for five minutes I visualize and feel my body filled with shimmering, healing light. I imagine myself full of vitality and energy. I picture myself in the future, healthy and vibrantly alive. I take action steps toward that end, which include eating healthy foods, taking herbs and supplements, exercising, and listening to meditation tapes that raise my vibration. Another action step I'm taking toward believing I'm healed and have a future ahead of me...I'm buying new clothes! This is the reality I'm choosing to focus on and manifest.

I can't help but wonder sometimes if my fear of cancer was a focus that created it in me. That's what the law of attraction would say. But if so, I reassure myself that I'm in good company. Many people on a spiritual path like I am, people who were living a health and spirit-oriented life, nonetheless got cancer. Including Wayne Dyer, who once wrote, "What you really, really want, you'll get. And what you really, really don't want, you'll also get. What you are focused on in your mind is what you attract." Larry Dossey, in his book *Healing Words*, presents a long list of saints who died of cancer, Krishnamurti among them. Even Jane Roberts, despite healing advice from Seth, died at the age of 55 from a crippling autoimmune disease.

On the ego level, this could seem like a failure. Yet, who knows what our souls are up to. I'm deeply aware of my souls passionate agenda to learn and grow and evolve my consciousness. My ego's agenda is to have fun and avoid suffering. I believe that ultimately soul's agenda trumps ego's agenda. In my case, that's the result anyway; and in accordance with the law of attraction, the result will ALWAYS show you your strongest intention. My soul wants to wake up as much as possible in this lifetime, and I am now awake much of the time. Therefore, cancer has been a means to that end, (instead of a mean end.)

Jane Roberts also wrote in her letter to me, "Love the dusk and the dawn. Be thankful for this life." I am thankful for this life, and thankful for this wake-up call that has made my life richer and more vivid. I like the reality that I've created. (At least my SOUL does—my ego is sometimes not too crazy about it!)

How about you? Do you like the reality you've created? If not, you can change it. You are the boss of your own reality! "You are given the gift of the gods; you create your reality according to your beliefs; yours is the creative energy that makes your world; there are no limitations to the self except those you believe in."–(Seth)

## 59

# COMPASSIONATE WITNESS
(September 21, 2011)

When I was in my early twenties, I read an article in Parade Magazine about Liza Minnelli, who had just emerged from rehab. Something she said in that article has stayed with me all these years. It was very simple, yet so vastly profound that it helped change my life forever. She said that she was developing a new relationship with herself and throughout the day would check in asking, "How are you doing honey?"

That blew my mind! The thought that I could talk to myself that way opened up a whole new way of being with myself. I started checking in with myself and calling myself "honey' and 'sweetheart'. Gradually, over time, the critical voice that was always beating me up became a loving voice. My chronic, internal judge was being replaced by my Compassionate Witness. This is an on-going process that continues to this day.

In my forties I fortified the voice of my Compassionate Witness by doing a two-year training in Hakomi, a healing, therapeutic approach that brings mindfulness, curiosity, and loving presence to whatever is present. Strengthening the energy of presence was building a mighty muscle that would carry me through tough times.

I flex that muscle now whenever I'm haunted by horror thoughts of possible cancer carnage—I take deep breaths and become very present. This invites in my Compassionate Witness, who says, "I know that you feel scared right now honey. Let yourself feel it." I reassure myself that when and if that time comes, I will be present with what's present, breathing into it, fully feeling and facing it, putting on my Big Soul panties and dealing with it. (And, if it gets too bad...LOTS of powerful, kick-ass painkillers...because saint I ain't!)

I know that healing happens in the light of awareness. The glue that binds our painful feelings and patterns together is soluble in awareness, which is much like water: "Nothing in the world is as soft and yielding as water; yet for dissolving the hard and inflexible, nothing can surpass it."-(Lao Tzu) Awareness is very potent stuff!

When I bring my Compassionate Witness to everything I think, do and feel, something astonishing happens...I gradually BECOME more the witness than the thing that I'm witnessing! When I bring all my shadows into the light, I become whole, welcoming every part of me to the party. My Compassionate Witness throws a great party! Every shadow, every guest who shows up (and they are quite a motley cast of characters!) is welcomed with open arms. Even the biggest shadow of them all...death.

Facing our death is something we're all going to have to do eventually—it is the big fat elephant in the room. Buddha said, "Just as the elephant's footprint is the biggest footprint on the jungle floor, death is the biggest teacher. Death or Yama Raja, death personified, drove me to the peace beyond birth and death."

I want to be in that peace beyond birth and death; therefore, I'm intent on facing my fear of death, and death itself, and making friends with it. That way I am embracing it, rather than bracing against it. Leonard Cohen wrote, "If you don't become the ocean you'll be seasick every day." When I come into harmony with all that floats and flounders about in my ocean, I am at peace.

Since what I resist persists, I'm hoping that now that

I'm no longer resisting, maybe death won't be persisting! Not any time soon anyway. Hopefully, I'll have many more years to practice being fully present with my fears about the big "C" and the big "D"—bringing me more into union with the big ME, my true oceanic self!

Byron Katie said: "Life is simple. Everything happens for you, not to you. Everything happens at exactly the right moment, neither too soon nor too late. You don't have to like it…it's just easier if you do." With the loving support of my Compassionate Witness, my greatest intention is to face whatever happens, and all my feelings about what happens, with an open mind, an open heart, and open arms.

Do you have a Compassionate Witness? There is no better traveling companion on life's journey…it will help you get through ANYTHING!

# 60

# CHAOS IS AN 'OBSTACLE' ILLUSION
(October 9, 2011)

In my first newsletter I asked the question, "What wants to be born into my life?" Now, two-and-a-half years later I have my answer—I have been reborn into a new life, a new way of being, a higher version of myself. I can see now that I had so many fears jamming me up, creating a stagnation that kept me from fully stretching into this life. Cancer was the chaos that stirred my stagnation into the birth of a more vibrant aliveness. As Bob Dylan sang, "He not busy being born, is busy dying." I'm now busy being born!

For me, cancer instigated a total cleanse of my body, emotions, and spirit, removing toxins, blocks, and beliefs that had kept life from flowing through me fully. I have come more into harmony with myself and now appreciate every part of my body...and I mean EVERY part. I never thought I'd be applauding voluminous bowel movements, but I am! They are so beautiful to me! They let me know that the obstruction that was there before hasn't grown back! All systems are clear and flowing!

I'm seeing that illness can be a rousing call to wholeness and more vibrancy. What seems like chaos and disaster is actually all part of an innate intelligence and drive towards greater creativity and a higher order of being.

This is beautifully illustrated in Cymatics, the study of sound and vibration in which the surface of a plate is vibrated and a thin layer of particles on the plate resonate with the vibration, eventually forming a cohesive pattern. As the frequency rises, chaos ensues—the particles go haywire, into total disarray! Then, at a certain point the particles spontaneously reorganize once again, forming an even more intricate, symmetrical, interconnected, mandala-like pattern. This process repeats itself each time the frequency increases; disintegration is followed by re-integration and a higher order of harmony and coherence ensues.

I believe this same process happens in illness and other life challenges—chaos is a purposeful response to stagnation and a prelude to a higher state of being. However, the success of this transition depends on how we perceive these challenges; when upheavals happen it can either seem like the death of us, or an opportunity to grow and raise our game to a higher level. Once I see that chaos is just an 'obstacle illusion', I stop kicking and screaming and resisting, and I come into harmony with this process of rebirth. I can then ride the spiral of my personal growth upwards, saying, "Oh boy, another growth opportunity!"

To determine our physical health, a doctor checks our vital signs. What I've learned is to determine my emotional and spiritual health by checking my vitality signs: am I fully engaged and living a creative life, facing and integrating shadows, fulfilling my life purpose? If so, I don't need to create chaos. But if chaos comes again, I will stay with it, learn from it, and ride it out, knowing that it is all part of elevating my life to a higher level of being. Nietzsche said, "You need chaos in your soul to give birth to a dancing star." When stuck in stagnation we are stirred and steered onward and upward to become the stars that we truly are!

Is your life in chaos right now? Congratulations! Something magnificent is about to be born into form!

# EPILOQUE:
# AMAZING SURPRISES AHEAD!

"Psss-s-s-s-t-t, S-h-h-h-h-h-h! Around the bend, in the unseen, arising from the very uncertainties that may now seem to taunt you, there are some amazing surprises, awesome twists, and spellbinding coincidences about to emerge that you can't even now imagine." This was the perfect Note from the Universe from Mike Dooley that I recently received. It's been over a year since I went through my 6-week radiation and chemo treatment for my recurrent uterine cancer. During that time I was deeply immersed in the misery of nausea, weakness, and the dismal awareness that the chances of the grueling treatment working were slim to none. It was difficult to imagine that a year later I'd still be here…thriving!

With time possibly limited, I was motivated this year to deeply immerse myself in the present moment, savoring it like delicious candy, and to my great delight, time has stretched like taffy into a sweet eternal Nooow! The quality of time has literally changed me. I don't just know, I *feel* that right now is all there is. Whenever my mind races into a feared future, I say "Whoa Nelly!" and take deep slow breaths, bringing my mind back to the bounty of this nourishing present moment. This is a great treasure I have found!

Another great treasure I've discovered on this journey is the priority of focusing on the healing energy of love. For the rest of my life, however long that is, love is what I want to create and where I want to dwell. How much I have loved in this life is something I believe I take with me when I go.

I have also lasered into living my life on purpose, getting

on with what I came here to do—writing from my heart and soul and sharing it with others. It is a treasure beyond measure to think that I can be of service in this way.

I have learned to not sweat the small stuff, but instead to celebrate the big stuff, like the present moment, love, and living a purposeful life. What a bountiful banquet I have found myself at! I couldn't have known a year ago when things seemed so dire, that a more vibrant, meaningful, luscious life was about to unfold.

I don't know for certain if I'm cured, but what I do know is that I am healed in the truest sense of word. The word 'heal' literally means 'to be whole', and because of this journey, I am whole—I am in harmony with my emotions, my body, and my spirit. I am wholly, vibrantly alive. I have surrendered to what is, trusting that I am right where I'm supposed to be.

Can you remember times when things looked bleak, but turned out even better than you could imagine? When we hang in there, twists and turns and coincidences present themselves, and our life miraculously goes from sucky to succulent, from yucky to YUM! No matter how things may seem, be open for surprises and miracles! Life is an amazing adventure filled with growth opportunities galore! While we are still here, let's go for it!

www.ingramcontent.com/pod-product-compliance
Lightning Source LLC
Chambersburg PA
CBHW050117280326
41933CB00010B/1139